MCQs in APHERESIS MEDICINE

AF679099

LEAD AUTHOR AND COORDINATOR:
DR. Y. SWAPNA

EDITORS:
DR. AIKAJ JINDAL,
DR. ASEEM TIWARI,
DR. SANGEETA PATHAK

notionpress.com
INDIA · SINGAPORE · MALAYSIA

Copyright © Dr. Y. Swapna 2026
All Rights Reserved.

ISBN
Paperback 979-8-90362-339-6
Hardcase 979-8-90392-652-7

This book has been published with all efforts taken to make the material error-free after the consent of the author. However, the author and the publisher do not assume and hereby disclaim any liability to any party for any loss, damage, or disruption caused by errors or omissions, whether such errors or omissions result from negligence, accident, or any other cause.

While every effort has been made to avoid any mistake or omission, this publication is being sold on the condition and understanding that neither the author nor the publishers or printers would be liable in any manner to any person by reason of any mistake or omission in this publication or for any action taken or omitted to be taken or advice rendered or accepted on the basis of this work. For any defect in printing or binding the publishers will be liable only to replace the defective copy by another copy of this work when available.

This book contains material created with the assistance of artificial intelligence tools. The author has curated, edited, and shaped the final content and the cover design, ensuring originality and creative expression. The copyright belongs solely to the Lead author.

FOREWORD

I am delighted to write this foreword for MCQs in Apheresis Medicine, a timely and thoughtfully curated resource compiled by a dedicated clinician from our Blood Centre. Apheresis medicine has emerged as a vital subspecialty at the intersection of transfusion services, critical care, haematology, oncology, and transplantation. With its expanding clinical applications—from therapeutic plasma exchange to cellular collections—there is a growing need for structured learning tools that translate complex concepts into practical knowledge. This book admirably addresses that need through a focused, question-based format that encourages active learning and self-assessment. The MCQ approach adopted in this volume is particularly valuable for postgraduate trainees, transfusion medicine specialists, and practicing clinicians alike. By combining core principles with clinically relevant scenarios, the author has created a resource that not only supports examination preparation but also reinforces evidence-based decision-making in day-to-day practice. What stands out is the clarity of presentation and the breadth of topics covered, with clear delineation of chapters, reflecting both academic rigor and real-world experience from the Blood Centre. Such contributions are essential in strengthening capacity building in transfusion and apheresis services, especially in resource-diverse healthcare settings.

At Cancer Institute (WIA), Chennai, we strongly believe in fostering academic excellence alongside compassionate, patient-centred care. Publications like this exemplify that commitment by empowering healthcare professionals with accessible, high-quality educational material that ultimately benefits patients. I congratulate every author on their commendable effort and am confident that this book will serve as a practical companion for students and clinicians, and as a meaningful addition to the growing body of literature in apheresis medicine.

I wish this work every success and wide readership.

DR KALPANA BALAKRISHNAN
CEO & MEDICAL DIRECTOR
CANCER INSTITUTE (WIA)

CANCER INSTITUTE (WIA) CHENNAI 600 020

PREFACE

Apheresis in Transfusion Medicine is an emerging clinically oriented speciality. There is a great need for solid decision-making and a strong conceptual grasp due to the growing indications in haematology, neurology, nephrology, critical care, and transplant medicine. The Post graduate students and the practitioners face some difficulties to bring the evidence-based guidelines into clinical practice as apheresis involves and revolves around physiology, pathology and technology.

The aim of this book is to address the gap between the theory and practical aspects through a concentrated, exam oriented and clinical approach. The multiple-choice questions (MCQ) style is deliberately chosen to highlight the scope for active learning, self-evaluation and collection of important concepts. The analytical thinking reinforces the genuine clinical scenarios.

The basic concepts, primitive and advance technologies, equipment, vascular access, anticoagulation, safety of donors and patients, therapeutic apheresis indications and procedural troubleshoots and latest applications are covered in the book. The book is helpful for both exams and routine clinical decision-making since the questions are in line with accepted standards and current practice. The physicians of transfusion medicine, haematology, and related fields can benefit. It also could help for short review and serve as refresher for the students preparing for specialized exams.

In order to maintain high acadcmic standards, a team of eminent national and international faculty as editors and dedicated contributors have worked together to compile this book. I thank every individual who has been part of this academic endeavour. Learning science and medicine is a continuous journey.

Dr. Y. Swapna
Lead Author & coordinator

Editors*

Dr. Aikaj Jindal,
Senior Consultant and Head, Department of Transfusion Medicine,
Mohandai Oswal Hospital, Ludhiana, Punjab

Dr. Aseem Tiwari,
Senior Director, Transfusion Medicine (Blood Center),
Medanta-the Medicity Hospital, Gurugram

Dr. Sangeeta Pathak,
Director & Head - Transfusion Services,
Max Super speciality Hospital, Delhi

**The names of the editors are arranged according to alphabetical order*

Authors

Dr. Y Swapna
Dr. Indira S Puthran
Dr. KM Haripriya
Dr. P Sunantha
Dr. Shahida Noushad
Dr. Priyanka C Gopinathan

CONTENTS

Chapter 1

HISTORY, EVOLUTION INSTRUMENTATION AND PRINCIPLES OF APHERESIS

Dr. Sunantha and Dr. Swapna

Q1. The word plasmapheresis was coined by

1. Abel et al
2. Dr. Edwin Cohn
3. Dr. Carl Gustav
4. Allen Latham

Q2. Which of the following is true regarding the scientists and their contributions?

1. John Abel, Clement Rowntree, and Leonard Turner - performed the first manual plasmapheresis on a dog model to separate plasma from whole blood
2. Carl Gustaf Patrik De Laval- developed the process for separating blood plasma into its individual components, which was crucial for saving lives during World War I
3. George Judson and Dr. Emil Freireich- were involved in construction of steam turbines and milk dairy
4. Dr. Edwin Cohn- developed the latham bowl

Q3. Which among the following is true in the History of apheresis?

1. *Hippocrates* proposed in 400 BC that proper balance of the four bodily fluids is important for proper health of the human being and that evidence of misbalance is disease
2. The earliest continuous flow centrifugation device was created by Swedish scientist Carl Gustaf Patrik de Laval, who *patented* it as a centrifugal milk-cream separator
3. De Laval and Cohn are regarded as the *founding fathers* of the modern practice of apheresis science and medicine
4. All of the above

Q4. Identify the Scientist:

1. Dr. Carl Gustav Fig I-1, John J Abel Fig I-2
2. John J Abel Fig I-1, Dr. Carl Gustav Fig I-2
3. Dr. Carl Gustav Fig I-1, Dr. Edwin J Cohn Fig I-2
4. John J Abel Fig I-1, Dr. Edwin J Cohn Fig I-2

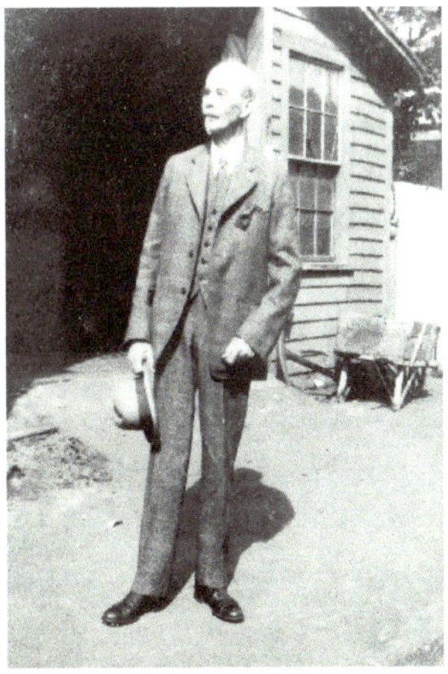

Fig I-1 Image-CCBY 4.0 (Original caption available in Answer key)

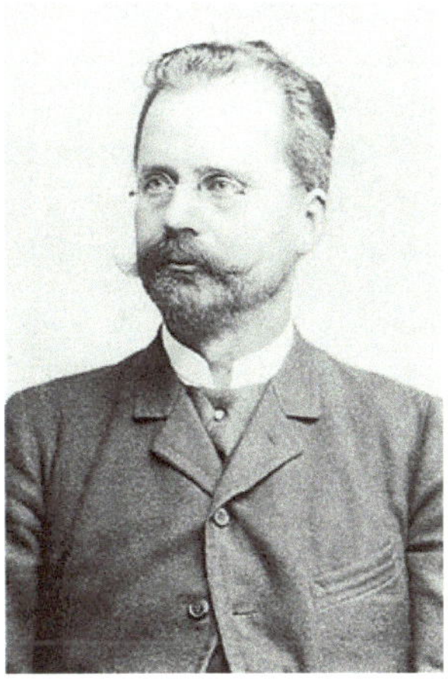

Fig I-2 Image - CCBY 4.0 (Original caption available in Answer key)

Q5. Which of the following is false regarding the development timeline of equipment?
1. Cohn fractionation was patented in 1951
2. Latham bowl was designed in 1952
3. COBE Labs Inc was founded in 1964
4. NCI-IBM 2990 was released for field trial in 1952

Q6. Which among the following is true with respect to modern apheresis equipment?
1. IBM engineer George T. Judson and Dr. Emil Freireich worked closely together to develop the first apheresis system at the National Cancer Institute
2. The first blood cell separator based on centrifugation was invented and it segregated leukocytes based on density in venous blood for the first time
3. This device also made it possible to extract cells selectively while giving the donor back the rest of the blood components
4. All of the above

Q7. Which among the following is true regarding filtration Techniques?
1. Willem Johan Kolff presented the first hemo-dialysis machine (artificial kidney) in 1943
2. Plasma was filtered with the use of animal-derived membrane
3. Semipermeable filtration membranes based on this principle are used for apheresis procedures
4. All of the above

Q8. Which among the following is false in the timeline?
1. Hemonetics model 30 was released for TPE and cell separation in 1973
2. Fenwall Celltrifuge II was released for TPE and cell separation in1976
3. IBM 2997 single chanel system was introduced in 1977
4. Fenwal / Baxter CS 3000 was introduced in1977

Q9. Which of the following is false regarding the procedure of apheresis equipment?
1. Fenwal / Baxter CS 3000 used 8080 microprocessor chips to prime and test the tubing before the procedure
2. Fenwal / Baxter CS 3000 used 8080 microprocessor chips to respond to the signals from an optical monitor to make the separation more efficient
3. IBM 2997 Single Channel system had a rectangular cross section formed into a loop, whole blood entered through the channel via a single port and was separated by centrifugal force
4. None of the above

Q10. Which of the following is true in the evolution of the instruments?
1. Hemonetics model V50 was released for TPE and cell separation in 1981
2. Fenwal / Baxter PS-400 was introduced for plasma separation in 1980
3. Fresenius AS- 104 was introduced in 1987
4. COBE Spectra was introduced in1987

Q11. Which of the following is false regarding the centrifuges?
1. The concept for the sealless blood-processing centrifuge that was used in CS 3000 and celltrifuge II began in January 1973 (nonrotating electrical connection technique)
2. The Adams principle was applied to the Fenwal Elutramatic blood washer as well as the Aminco Celltrifuge and was called the "jump rope" technique
3. It was aimed to eliminate the troublesome rotating seal
4. None of the above

Q12. Which of the following is true about Centry TPE – flat Membrane Plasma Separation?
1. It is used as a flat parallel plate membrane for plasma separation
2. It was the first membrane separation filter approved by the United States FDA and was as effective as centrifugal methods
3. Membrane plasma separation is biocompatible and has a pore size that will allow the passage of all plasma constituents
4. All of the above

Q13. Which of the following is false with respect to IBM 2997/COBE Spectra?
1. The "*floppy bag*" laminated channel looking like a cross section of the channel of the 2990 bowl; was wrapped in an arc around the centre of rotation and included in IBM 2997/COBE Spectra
2. Earlier evaluation of this equipment indicated that *acceptable* plasma separation could be attained with it
3. *Differential* cell separation however, could not be achieved with this instrument
4. None of the above

Q14. Which of the following is true regarding substance characteristics and associated removal methods?
1. Distribution volume and compartment have a role when removal methods are by diffusion, filtration and adsorption
2. Charge of the substance has a role when removal is by means of adsorption
3. Plasma exchange removes soluble substances only from the intravascular compartment
4. All of the above

Q15. Which of the following is not true regarding depletion of a substance due to metabolic characteristics?
1. The substance's net clearance is determined by equilibration across body fluid compartments
2. As the substances redistribute intravascularly for elimination, those with a large extravascular distribution will be eliminated more quickly
3. Rapid rebound results from the faster synthesis of substances with shorter half-lives
4. More frequent TPE is required for removal of substances with shorter half-lives

Q16. Which of the following is true regarding the catabolism of proteins?
1. The Fractional Catabolic Rate of IgM is 18%; Transcapillary escape rate is 1-2%
2. The Fractional Catabolic Rate of IgG is 6.7%; Transcapillary escape rate is 3%
3. The Fractional Catabolic Rate of Albumin is 10%; Transcapillary escape rate is 5-6%
4. All of the above

Q17. Which of the following is true regarding the serum concentration of proteins?
1. The concentration of IgM in normal serum/plasma is 0.9 mg/ml
2. The concentration of IgG in normal serum/plasma is 12.1 mg/ml
3. The concentration of albumin in normal serum/plasma is 42 mg/ml
4. All of the above

Q18. The proportion of a substance removed from the entire body during a single session of therapeutic plasma exchange (TPE) depends largely on its metabolic characteristics, particularly its intravascular distribution. Based on these metabolic features, which protein would be expected to be removed to the greatest extent during a single TPE procedure?
1. Albumin (40% intravascular)
2. IgG (45% intravascular)
3. IgM (76% intravascular)
4. Fibrinogen (80% intravascular)

Q19. Which of the following is true regarding the size and the specific gravity of the blood component?
1. Platelet diameter 3µm , Specific gravity 1.040
2. Red cell diameter 9 µm , Specific gravity 1.093-1.096
3. Lymphocyte diameter 12 µm , Specific gravity 1.060
4. Granulocyte diameter 10 µm , Specific gravity 1.087-.1.099

Q20. Ideal target molecule characteristics for therapeutic plasma exchange are all except
1. Identified etiologic agent or toxic substance
2. High molecular mass
3. Slow rate of formation and low turnover
4. High volume of distribution

Q21. Which of the following mechanisms is false for removal of substances?
1. Hemodialysis (Diffusion clearance) - For small molecules(<500Da)
2. Hemofiltration (Convection Clearance)- For small and middle molecules(<500Da-15000Da)
3. Therapeutic Plasma exchange - For large molecules (15000->150000Da)
4. None of the above

Q22. Which of the following is true regarding Immunoglobulin G removal by plasma exchange?
1. Equilibration between the extravascular and intravascular compartments and the production of new immunoglobulin G are the causes of the intertreatment rise
2. Immunoglobulin G (IgG) synthesis, its long half-life (22 days), and its low daily turnover are linked to the majority of immunological complex illnesses
3. Circulating IgG levels will drop to 16%–20% of the baseline level after six doses with TPE every other day
4. All of the above

Q23. Which of the following is true in Elutriation Techniques?

1. In this technique, there is use of two opposite forces namely the centrifugal force and the flow of plasma
2. In the product collection line, a specific elutriation chamber is placed in which the heavier cells are pushed to the centrifuge wall
3. A second separation of the blood cells based on the size of these cells is forced simultaneously, with an opposite force caused by a fluid flow
4. All of the above

Q24. All of the following are true regarding Elutriation in apheresis techniques except

1. Is used to achieve leukoreduction of the collection of specific mononuclear cells (lymphocytes and monocytes)
2. Is used to reduce the donor's platelet loss due to the apheresis procedure
3. The sequence of the various blood components with elutriation techniques is plasma—platelets—erythrocytes—lymphocytes— Haematopoietic Progenitor Cells (HPCs) (when present)—granulocytes—monocytes
4. None of the above

Q25. Which of the following is false regarding the mechanisms of TPE?

1. The main targeted pathogenic substances with TPE are antibodies
2. TPE acts by altering the ratio of T helper type-1 and type-2 cells in the peripheral blood, which mediates with antibody-secreting B-cells to inhibit antibody production
3. TPE can also elevate the response of cells to immunosuppressive agents and also removes immune mediated cells from circulation
4. None of the above

Q26. Which of the following is false when procedures are done by Terumo BCT Trima Accel?

1. Collects platelets with Extra Corporeal Volume- 196 ml
2. Collects RBC/Plasma and Plasma only with Extra Corporeal Volume- 182 ml
3. Uses leukoreduction filter and is single access system
4. None of the above

Q27. Which of the following is true regarding Acousto fluidic-based strategy for therapeutic apheresis (ATAS)?

1. This strategy was proposed to meet the needs of therapeutic apheresis procedures that involves patients with limited blood volume
2. The ATAS strategy uses an acousto fluidic microchip to ensure blood cells, platelets, and plasma are separated in a continuous and stable manner
3. Cellular components of blood are separated and transferred into the sheath fluid while antibodies remain in the plasma component due to their solubility
4. All of the above

Q28. Which of the following with respect to the SONOFLOW series is false?

1. Hybrid ultrasound sensor SONOFLOW CO.56 Pro V 2.0 is used for flow-bubble detection
2. They are designed for medical equipments like cardiopulmonary bypass, extracorporeal membrane oxygenation (ECMO), organ transport and dialysis machines
3. They are used in apheresis equipments
4. They are not used to detect flow rates

Q29. Which of the following is true regarding AI in therapeutic apheresis?

1. ChatGPT-4o, o1-preview, and Claude 3.5 Sonnet (New) are some of the AI models under research
2. The integration of artificial intelligence (AI) and machine learning (ML) in Apheresis technology can help the development of more sophisticated and personalized apheresis procedures
3. Computer code generated by ChatGPT-4o is being evaluated for its full function in both Python and Colaboratory
4. All of the above

Q30. What is the purpose of Plasmat Futura?

1. It is a device used to perform Heparin-induced Extracorporeal Low Density Lipoprotein precipitation- H.E.L.P. apheresis
2. It is helpful in patients with familial hypercholesterolemia and hyperlipoproteinemia (a)
3. It is useful in patients suffering from hyperfibrinogenemia and transplant vasculopathy
4. All of the above

ANSWERS

Q1. Ans(1)
In 1914, Abel, Rowntree, and Turner coined the term plasmaphaeresis, derived from the Greek word *aphairesis*, meaning withdrawal. Their initial efforts aimed to alleviate symptoms following bilateral nephrectomy in dogs. Despite the association of these experiments with fatalities (attributable to excessive bleeding and hemorrhage), the enhancement in the clinical condition of the successfully treated animals was remarkable. The term apheresis has been broadly used to denote the separation of blood into its constituents, extracting/collecting one component, and reinfusing the remaining.

Dr. Edwin J. Cohn: Edwin J. Cohn (1892-1953). Cohn served as a professor of biological chemistry at Harvard Medical School and was among the pioneers in applying fundamental physical, chemical concepts to the study of amino acids and proteins. During World War II, Cohn oversaw research initiatives aimed at developing techniques for the separation of human plasma into various components for clinical application in the Armed Forces.

Dr. Carl Gustav Patrick de Laval (9 May 1845 – 2 February 1913) was a Swedish engineer and inventor renowned for his significant advancements in the construction of steam turbines and centrifugal separation machinery for the dairy industry.

Allen Latham - The 1991 Norwich Native Son was Allen "Jack" Latham, Jr. The blood-separation technology developed by Jack Latham and his associates transformed transfusion techniques. It has enhanced the efficacy of platelet donations and the capacity to eliminate toxins from the blood. Physicians can either collect components for transfusion or extract substances from a patient that are harmful.

Q2. Ans(1)

Q3. Ans(4)

Q4. Ans(2)
Figure I-1. Portrait of J.J. Abel (reproduced). Courtesy of Well come Library, London. (22) 1929. Licensed under Creative Commons Attribution 4.0 International (CC BY 4.0), via Wikimedia Commons.
Figure I-2. *Gustaf de Laval* [Internet image] reproduced. Wikimedia Commons; Public domain. [cited 2026 Feb 12].(23)

Q5. Ans(4)
NCI-IBM 2990 was released for field trial in1966

Q6. Ans(4)

Q7. Ans(4)

Q8. Ans(4)
Fenwal / Baxter CS 3000 was introduced- 1979

Q9. Ans(4)

Q10. Ans(4)

Q11. Ans(4)

Q12. Ans(4)

Q13. Ans(4)

Q14. Ans(4)
Plasma proteins are produced which is determined by synthetic rate (S); proteins are degraded and/or removed from the plasma and it is determined by the fractional catabolic rate, or FCR(both the rates are equal). In contrast to the extraction of plasma from the intravascular compartment through plasma exchange, S, FCR, and the migration of solutes within compartments are in equilibrium and maintain a steady state, occurring at a significantly slower pace.

Q15. Ans(2)
Substances that have a significant extravascular distribution will be eliminated at a slower rate, as they need to redistribute within the intravascular space before they can be removed.

Q16. Ans(4)

Q17. Ans(4)

Q18. Ans(4)

Q19. Ans(1)

Q20. Ans(4)

Q21. Ans(4)
The molecular weights (expressed in kilodaltons) are indicated as outlined. The sieving coefficients, which are established by the ratio of solute concentrations between the filtrate and blood sides of the membrane for larger molecules, are almost equal to one, for proteins with molecular weights ranging from that of albumin to B-lipoprotein (2,400,000 Da), and may extend to the weight of cryoglobulins (900,000 Da). At the higher end of the spectrum, the exclusion of platelets (1–2 µm) and the rejection of proteins with extremely high molecular weights (3,000,000 Da) are noted characteristics.

Q22. Ans(4)

Q23. Ans(4)

Q24. Ans(4)

Q25. Ans(4)

Q26. Ans(4)

Q27. Ans(4)

Q28. Ans(4)

Q29. Ans(4)

Q30. Ans(4)

REFERENCES

1. Burgstaler EA, Winters JL. Basic principles of apheresis and the collection of bloodcomponents by apheresis: Simon TL, Gehrie EA, McCullough J, Roback JD, Snyder EL. Rossi'sPrinciples of Transfusion Medicine. 6th ed. Hoboken (NJ): Wiley-Blackwell; 2022.p.251.
2. Berger M. Immunoglobulin products: Simon TL, Gehrie EA, McCullough J, RobackJD, Snyder EL. Rossi's Principles of Transfusion Medicine. 6th ed. Hoboken (NJ):Wiley-Blackwell; 2022.p.238.
3. Brunker AR, Pagano BM. Therapeutic apheresis: plasma processing: Simon TL, GehrieEA, McCullough J, Roback JD, Snyder EL. Rossi's Principles of Transfusion Medicine.6th ed. Hoboken (NJ): Wiley-Blackwell; 2022.p.259.
4. Pohar M, Hansson N. Between two stools? Pharmacologists nominated for Nobel prizes in"physiology or medicine" and "chemistry" 1901–1950 with a focus on John Jacob Abel(1857–1938). Naunyn-Schmiedeberg's Arch Pharmacol. 2021;394(3):503-513.
5. Freireich EJ, Judson G, Levin RH. Separation and collection of leukocytes. Cancer Res. 1965;25(9):1516–20.
6. Winters JL, editor. Apheresis: principles and practice. 4th ed.Vol.1, Therapeutic Apheresis. Bethesda, MD:AABB; 2020
7. C. Elena Cervantes, Bloch EM, C. John Sperati. Therapeutic Plasma Exchange: Core Curriculum 2023. 2023 Feb 1;81(4):475–92.
8. McLeod BC, Szczepiorkowski ZM, Weinstein R, Winters JL, editors. Apheresis: Principles and Practice. 3rd ed. Bethesda, MD: AABB Press; 2010.
9. Williams ME, Balogun RA. Principles of Separation: Indications and Therapeutic Targets for Plasma Exchange. Clinical Journal of the American Society of Nephrology [Internet]. 2014 Jan 7;9(1):181–90. Available from: https://cjasn.asnjournals.org/content/9/1/181
10. Kozanoglu I *Problem Solving in Apheresis Medicine*, Switzerland: Springer Nature; 2024
11. Hu Y, Yang H, Fu S, Wu J (2022) Therapeutic plasma exchange: for Cancer patients. Cancer Manag Res 14:411–425
12. The Immunomodulatory Role of Therapeutic Plasma Exchange in Peripheral Nervous System and Neuromuscular Diseases. 1 [Internet]. 2017 Feb 2 [cited 2024 Feb 10]; Available from: https://touchneurology.com/neuromuscular-diseases/journal-articles/
13. Zanatta E, Cozzi M, Marson P, Cozzi F. The role of plasma exchange in the management of autoimmune disorders. *Br J Haematol.* 2019;186(2):207–219.
14. Barlogie B, Alexanian R, Jagannath S (1992) Plasma Cell Dys crasias JAMA 268(20):2946–2951
15. Smith WJ. Blood Component Collection by Apheresis: Fung MK, Grossman BJ, HillyerCD, Westhoff CM. Technical manual. 18th ed. Bethesda (MD): AABB; 2014.p.174
16. Wu M, Ma Z, Xu X, Lu B, Gu Y, Yoon J, et al. Acoustofluidic-based therapeutic apheresis system. Nature Communications [Internet]. 2024 Aug 10 [cited 2025 Dec 11];15(1). Available from: https://pmc.ncbi.nlm.nih.gov/articles/PMC11316742/
17. USA. Apheresis – non-invasive fluid monitoring for medical technology[Internet]. Elmsford (NY): Sonotec USA; c2024 [cited 2026 Jan 25]. Available from:https://www.sonotecusa.com/products/non-invasive-fluid-monitoring/medtech/apheresis/
18. Anstey C, Ullman D, Su L, Su C, Siniard C, Simmons S, et al. The practical use of artificial intelligence in Transfusion Medicine and Apheresis. Transfusion and Apheresis Science. 2024; 63(6):104001.
19. Braun Ireland. Plasmat Futura [Internet]. Dublin: B. Braun Ireland; [cited 2026 Jan 25]. Available from: https://www.bbraun.ie/en/products/b0/plasmat-futura.html
20. Noiri E. and Hanafusa N., The Concise Manual of Apheresis Therapy. Tokyo: Springer Japan;2014
21. SONOFLOW CO.56 Pro V2.0 Technical Data Sheet Ultrasonic Flow-Bubble Sensor
22. Wellcome Library, London. *Portrait of J.J. Abel* [Internet]. Wikimedia Commons; [cited 2026 Feb 12]. Available from: https://commons.wikimedia.org/wiki/File:Portrait_of_J.J._Abel_Wellcome_M0016927.jpg. Licensed under Creative Commons Attribution 4.0 International (CC BY 4.0)
23. [cited 2026 Feb 12]. Available from: https://commons.wikimedia.org/wiki/File:GustafDeLaval.jpg. This work is in the public domain where copyright term is life + 70 years or fewer (Gustaf de Laval lived 1845–1913).

Chapter 2

GENERAL CONCEPTS

Dr. Swapna , Dr. Sunantha and Dr. Priyanka

Q1. Which of the following is true regarding Apheresis society?
1. Apheresis society was formed in 1982
2. Apheresis society was formed in 1992
3. Apheresis society was formed in 1999
4. Apheresis society was formed in 2002

Q2. McLeod's criteria are used to determine the success of Therapeutic Apheresis (TA) in a disease's treatment. Which of the following are the components?
1. The understanding of the disease pathogenesis facilitates a defined indication for TA
2. The abnormality is most likely to be corrected by TA
3. There is evidence that TA is clinically beneficial
4. All of the above

Q3. Which physical principle is utilized by all general-purpose blood cell separator devices currently in use?
1. Filtration
2. Centrifugation
3. Immunoadsorption
4. Electrophoresis

Q4. The following is true regarding ASFA (American Society for Apheresis) Guidelines except:
1. Since 1986, the ASFA Journal of Clinical Apheresis Special Issue Writing Committee has regularly issued guidelines regarding the application of therapeutic apheresis
2. The most recent update represents the ninth special issue, published in 2023, and is accessible for clinical application
3. The ninth special issue exclusively focuses on diseases that possess a substantial amount of documented evidence to support (or not to) the use of therapeutic apheresis
4. None of the above

Q5. Which of the following is true with respect to the Latest ASFA Guidelines?
1. The diseases and their therapies are organized into *category* and *grading* systems by ASFA
2. The category indicates the effectiveness and priority of apheresis in treating a disease, whereas the grading assesses the quality of evidence backing the use of apheresis for that disease
3. The ninth edition of the ASFA Guidelines features seven new fact sheets, nine new indications added to existing fact sheets, and eight modifications in the category for current indications
4. All of the above

Q6. Which of the following is false regarding ASFA Guidelines?
1. The committee needs at least ten examples published in peer-reviewed journals within the previous ten years, preferably by multiple groups, in order to satisfy the requirements for a new fact sheet
2. New fact sheets are added every four years
3. Fact sheets for 91 illnesses and ailments are included in the most recent edition of the Journal of Clinical Apheresis Special Issue. Additionally, the primary evaluation criterion for determining whether to conduct TA for a patient is the category of the disease
4. The Fourth Edition (2007) of ASFA introduces the idea of a fact sheet

Q7. Which of the following is true for categories in ASFA guidelines?
1. For ASFA category I indications, given that this designation indicates a *primary treatment modality*, it would be appropriate if the patient had no contraindications for the procedure, to proceed with the apheresis therapy
2. Disorders for which apheresis is *accepted as second line* therapy; either in standalone or in combination with other modes of treatment is category II

3. For ASFA category III indications, decision- making is more complex. The definition of this category indicates that "optimum *role* is *not* established" and "decision-making should be *individualized"* and for ASFA category IV indications, as the published evidence indicates that the apheresis procedure is *ineffective or harmful*, the procedure should not be performed
4. All of the above

Q8. ASFA adopted a grading recommendation suggested by
1. Guyatt G et al.
2. Connelly-Smith L et al.
3. Nadler SB et al.
4. Georges Guillain et al

Q9. All of the following are true in Therapeutic Plasma Exchange except
1. Membrane fractionation is one of the main techniques used for pathogen separation in apheresis therapy
2. The double filtration plasmapheresis (DFPP) has two (2) filters
3. The second filters in DFFP are available with same pore sizes
4. The pore size is selected based on the size needed to filter the specific pathogenic substance

Q10. Which of the following is true regarding the differences in plasmapheresis procedures by membranous and centrifugation methods?
1. Most centrifugal apheresis procedures require flow rates of 50–120 mL/min
2. Membrane apheresis procedures require flow rates of 150–200 mL/ min
3. Plasma extraction is 80% in cTPE and 30% in mTPE
4. All of the above

Q11. Which of the following is true regarding the complications in membranous and centrifugation methods?
1. Hemolysis is a complication often seen in membrane filtration
2. Increasing transmembrane pressure is a primary cause of hemolysis
3. Hemolysis does not occur in centrifugation method
4. All of the above

Q12. Which of the following factors are considered essential for the effectiveness of the membrane separation?
1. Transmembrane pressure (the difference in pressure between the blood and the filtrate sides of the membrane)
2. Haematocrit in the red cell fraction
3. Membrane separators are primed and operated conservatively in the beginning of the run in order to prevent excessive cell layering
4. All of the above

Q13. All of the following are true with respect to Therapeutic apheresis except
1. Plasma Exchange is used for removal of *pathogenic substances*
2. Plasma Exchange is used for *coagulation factor* supplementation
3. The efficacy of substance *removal* depends on molecular weight, distribution volume, compartment, production rate (half-life), electric charge, hydrophilic or hydrophobic properties, and specific gravity
4. The efficacy of substance removal from the blood is not determined by the apheresis devices used

Q14. Which of the following is true regarding bleeding and coagulation factors in Therapeutic Apheresis?
1. *Fresh frozen plasma* is used as the replacement fluid in patients with bleeding diathesis undergoing plasma exchange
2. Close monitoring of plasma *fibrinogen* level is necessary when filtration method is selected
3. A minimum interval of *24–48 h* between the filtration sessions is advised in order to support fibrinogen synthesis
4. All of the above

Q15. All of the following are true regarding hemo filters and plasma separators except
1. Hemofilters are used for molecules up to 20–30 kDa
2. Plasma separators are used in plasmapheresis to remove substances larger than albumin
3. The efficacy of filtration is not similar to that of dialysis with respect to per session or per hour removal of substances
4. None of the above

Q16. In Plasma Adsorption, all are true except

1. There are two types with respect to adsorption material design, it is woven as a *fabric* or formed into *beads* in one of them
2. In the other type, there are small molecule *ligands* that capture pathogenic substances which adhere to the *resin carrier*
3. Each subclass of IgG has a *different adsorptive capacity* in tryptophan conjugated column
4. *Molecular weight* differences do not determine the specificity for substance removal using adsorption

Q17. Which of the following is true for Central Venous Access (CVA)?

1. A *haemodialysis-compatible* catheter is required
2. CVA devices for apheresis procedures usually have two lumens, a shorter and mostly larger lumen for drawing (*red port*) and a longer lumen for returning blood (*blue port*)
3. These catheters are placed in the femoral vein or internal jugular vein and it is commonly designed to stay in them for *10–14 days*
4. All of the above

Q18. Which of the following is false regarding the venous access for apheresis?

1. Central Venous Catheters (CVC) placement in the cephalic, radial, ulnar veins can be used for apheresis
2. Implanted Intravascular Access Devices (PORT) are placed subcutaneously on the chest with the catheter further tunnelled into the distal superior vena cava or right atrium
3. Skin Tunnelled Catheters (Hickman Lines) are inserted through subclavian or jugular veins into the central circulation
4. Skin Tunnelled Catheters (Hickman Lines) are used for long term venous access (>30 days)

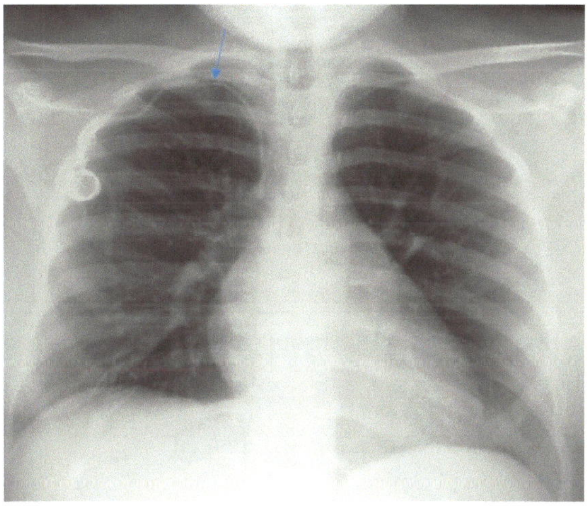

Fig II-1: Chest X-ray revealed Grade 2 luminal narrowing, consistent with pinch-off syndrome—a complication of subclavian catheter placement] reproduced from Correia MR et al. (35) 2025.
Licensed under Creative Commons Attribution 4.0 International (CC BY 4.0).

Q19. Which of the following is true regarding the image shown in Fig II-1?

1. *Pinch- off syndrome (POS)* is a rare and potentially life- threatening complication associated with implantable central venous catheters
2. POS is associated with *infraclavicular approach* of implantable catheters if the catheter is placed more medially
3. The catheter needs to be removed safely in order to avoid life- threatening complications such as *catheter fracture and embolization* of its fragments
4. All of the above

Q20. Which of the following is true with respect to Images Fig II-2 and Fig II-3?

1. Peripheral venous access device-short-with infusion (Fig II-2), Implanted venous access device (Fig II 3)
2. Non tunnelled central venous catheters (Fig II-2), Implanted venous access device (Fig II 3)
3. Peripheral venous access device- short-with infusion (Fig II-2), Non tunnelled central venous catheters (Fig II-3)
4. Non tunnelled central venous catheters (Fig II-2), Peripheral venous access device-short-with infusion (Fig II 3)

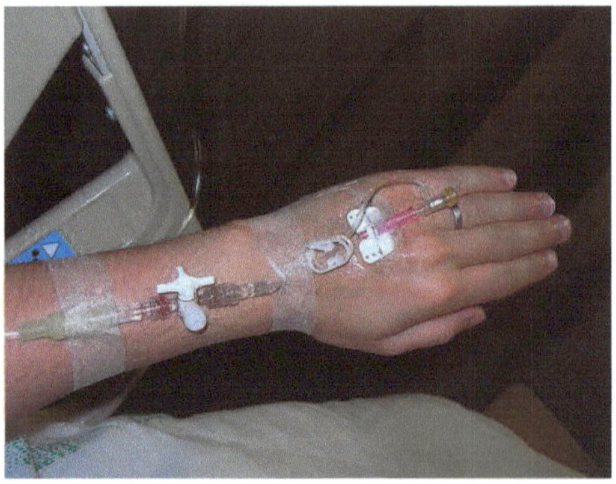

Fig II -2: Image reproduced from (Berry M) CCBY 4.0
(Original caption available in Answer key)

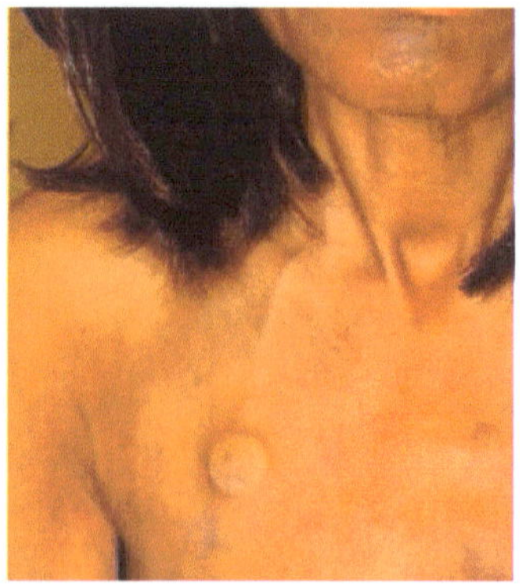

Fig II- 3: Image reproduced from (Una Smith) CCBY 4.0
(Original caption available in Answer key)

Q21. Which of the following is true in Peripheral Venous Access?

1. The median cubital veins are essential for access during blood draw and necessitate the use of 16–19 gauge steel or hard plastic needles, which are capable of withstanding the flow rates and negative pressure generated during an apheresis procedure
2. The blood flow rate achievable with a 17-gauge needle is approximately 80 mL/min or more, a 19–20 gauge needle allows for blood flow at around 60 mL/min
3. In instances where patients present with elevated haematocrit levels, typically exceeding 0.4, or in cases of hyperviscosity, it is advisable to utilize draw needles with larger gauges, such as a 16 gauge
4. All of the above

Q22. Which of the following is false for *identification* of Peripheral Venous Access (PVA)?

1. Near-infrared (NIR) imaging devices are used to help in the visual mapping of superficial veins for the purpose of assisting in PVA
2. These devices emit NIR light onto the skin, which is subsequently absorbed by deoxygenated hemoglobin
3. The vascular image is displayed on the patient's skin using visible green light, enhancing the capability to achieve PVA
4. None of the above

Q23. For selecting the Plasma Exchange dosage per session and session frequency, the following is required:

1. The distribution volume
2. The diffusion velocity between compartments
3. The production rate of the substance that needs to be removed
4. All of the above

Q24. The factors that influence the drug levels in plasma exchange are

1. Duration and frequency of apheresis procedures
2. Volume and rate of apheresis exchange
3. Methods of extracorporeal extraction used such as hemodialysis, hemoperfusion, hemofiltration, plasmapheresis
4. All of the above

Q25. Which of the following is true regarding distribution volume (V = Q/C)?

1. Distribution volume (V) can be expressed as V = Q/C, where Q is the total amount of the substance within the body and C is the concentration of the substance in the plasma
2. Drugs that exhibit significantly elevated volumes of distribution tend to have considerably greater concentrations in extravascular tissues compared to the vascular compartment; ie, they are not homogeneously distributed
3. Compounds that are confined to distribution within plasma, blood, the extracellular space, and in the overall water content of the body possess distribution volumes of 0.05, 0.07, 0.2, and 0.6 L/kg, respectively
4. All of the above

Q26. Which of the following with respect to distribution volume and diffusion velocity is false?

1. Substances with a distribution volume greater than 0.6 L/kg have good tissue penetration
2. The concentration at the end of therapy (C_T) is expressed as $C_T = C_0 e^{-KT/V}$, where K, T, V, and C_0 are clearance per unit of time, session duration, distribution volume, and the concentration at the beginning of therapy, respectively, which is applicable to a single compartment model
3. Repeat therapies effectively remove substances with a high diffusion velocity, while they are less effective for removing total amount of substances which have a slow velocity
4. None of the above

Q27. Which of the following fluids when used for replacement be responsible for the highest probability or risk of citrate toxicity during a plasma exchange procedure?

1. 0.9% normal saline
2. 5% albumin C
3. Lactated Ringer's solution
4. Plasma

Q28. Which of the following is false for citrate anticoagulation and calcium?

1. Donors often tolerate up to a 20% decline in ionized calcium levels
2. To stabilize ionized calcium levels, citrate delivery rates are arranged between 1.0 and 1.8 mg/kg/min
3. The most effective way to evaluate 'true' calcemia is through the direct measurement of serum-ionized calcium (Ca2+), (serum total calcium is influenced by serum proteins, albumin in particular)
4. None of the above

Q29. Hypocalcaemia management when serum ionized calcium <1.11 mmol/L is as follows

1. *1 gram* calcium gluconate IV when serum ionized calcium is 1.05–1.11 mmol/L; *2 grams* calcium gluconate IV when serum ionized calcium is 0.99–1.04 mmol/L
2. *3 grams* calcium gluconate IV when serum ionized calcium is 0.93–0.98 mmol/L; *4 grams* calcium gluconate IV when serum ionized calcium is <0.93 mmol/L
3. Evaluation of serum calcium levels is required after 4 hrs of replacement and not required in cases where *1 gram* calcium gluconate is the treatment
4. All of the above

Q30. During citrate anticoagulation in apheresis, ionized calcium levels decrease. Which physiological homeostatic mechanism is activated immediately in response to this reduction?

1. Increased secretion of thyroxine
2. Increased secretion of parathormone (PTH)
3. Decreased renal tubular reabsorption of calcium
4. Decreased intestinal absorption of calcium

Q31. What is the most common adverse effect observed during apheresis procedures that is attributable to transient hypocalcaemia caused by citrate anticoagulation?

1. Hypotension and bradycardia
2. Grand mal seizure
3. Mild perioral and/or peripheral paresthesias
4. Anaphylactic shock

Q32. If a patient undergoing apheresis reports mild, bothersome paresthesias (tingling or numbness) related to citrate toxicity, which of the following is the most appropriate first management step according to common practice guidelines?

1. Immediately infuse 10 mL of 10% calcium chloride intravenously
2. Administer oral calcium supplementation, such as a calcium-containing antacid
3. Reduce the total blood flow rate or the anticoagulant infusion rate (e.g., increase the whole blood: anticoagulant (WB:ACD) ratio)
4. Pause the procedure and place the patient in the Trendelenburg position

Q33. Monitoring citrate-induced ionized hypocalcemia is more challenging in young or sick children than in adults. Which set of symptoms is frequently noted in small children experiencing citrate toxicity, often in place of the mild perioral paresthesias common in adults?

1. Musculoskeletal pain, Bradycardia and hyperthermia
2. Confusion, muscle weakness and generalized seizure
3. Emesis (vomiting), abdominal pain, pallor, and/or hypotension
4. Facial edema, urticaria, and difficulty swallowing

Q34. Which of the following is false in calcium supplementation?

1. According to the *level of ionized calcium*, 10% calcium chloride is given as an infusion at a dose of 20 mg/kg (0.2 mL/kg) in more than 10 min
2. Citrate also chelates with *ionized magnesium (Mg++)*, causing ionized hypomagnesemia (presents with cardiovascular abnormalities as hypertension, arrhythmias, electrocardiogram changes)
3. The Mg++ level is monitored to ensure that magnesium replacement is done if cardiac symptoms do not improve with calcium replacement
4. None of the above

Q35. Why is it frequently recommended to omit the standard rinse-back step in therapeutic apheresis procedures for small infants (e.g.,10 kg)?

1. Rinse-back returns unnecessary donor red cells which increases the risk of iron overload
2. Rinse-back causes a full net fluid gain that could lead to severe volume overload in a small patient
3. Omission of rinse-back prevents the occurrence of ethylene oxide reactions from the tubing set
4. The residual red cell volume left in the circuit after omission is necessary for laboratory testing

Q36. Which of the following is false in anticoagulation by Heparin?

1. Heparin has a short half-life (23–168 min) and it is almost cleared during TPE
2. A bolus of 3000–5000 U is administered at the beginning of treatment, followed by a bolus of 1000 U/h when required
3. Heparin is the preferred anticoagulant in membrane filtration TPE
4. None of the above

Q37. Which among the following is false regarding Low molecular weight Heparin?

1. The discovery of Heparin was done incidentally, by a medical student J McLean in 1906
2. Low molecular weight heparin is often used for patients suffering from mild bleeding tendency
3. The dose of low molecular weight heparin usually is one-half the dose of heparin due to the *longer half-life of low molecular weight heparin*
4. None of the above

Q38. Which of the following is false regarding heparin as an anticoagulant in apheresis?

1. If heparin is administered as a simultaneous continuous infusion with citrate, WB: Citrate ratios are lowered
2. Continuous infusion (0.1-0.5 IU/kg/min) is given and it is important to maintain activated clotting time (ACT) at 180-210 seconds
3. Heparin can be added to ACD solution (5000 units to 500 mL ACD-A bag) and infused at a WB:AC ratio of 1:30
4. None of the above

Q39. Which of the following is true regarding heparin as an anticoagulant in apheresis?

1. Appropriate dosage of heparin is added to 0.9% normal saline
2. The delivery rate is ideally determined before the procedure
3. The inlet: AC (Anti-Coagulant) ratio is ideally set before the procedure
4. All of the above

Q40. The electrolyte disturbances associated with Plasma Exchange include all except

1. Hypocalcemia
2. Hypokalemia
3. Metabolic alkalosis
4. Hyperphosphatemia

Q41. A patient undergoing therapeutic apheresis develops symptoms of hypovolemia, including dizziness, light headedness, and hypotension. What is the recommended initial management strategy?

1. Increase the rate of replacement fluid infusion and continue the procedure
2. Halt the procedure, place the patient in the Trendelenburg position, and give a bolus of saline or colloid
3. Administer IV diphenhydramine and IV methylprednisolone
4. Immediately terminate the procedure and remove the vascular access

Q42. Which of the following is false during Therapeutic Apheresis in children with respect to hypotension?

1. Hypotension caused by hypovolemia is treated by administering bolus saline or colloid solutions
2. Priming the apheresis set with erythrocyte suspension is one of the methods to prevent hypovolemia in children
3. Hypotension is defined as systolic blood pressure at <45 mmHg in children under 4 years of age, <75 mmHg in children aged 5–8 years, <85 mmHg in children aged 9–12 years, and <95 mmHg in adolescents
4. None of the above

Q43. Which of the following is false regarding Catheter Insertion?

1. The catheter is inserted in Femoral/Subclavian/Internal jugular veins for Therapeutic apheresis
2. The right internal jugular is the commonly preferred venous insertion because the left internal jugular has a low blood flow due to inhibition caused by the tight angle to the right heart ventricle
3. Arterial puncture is noted in 3–15% of central venous access procedures
4. None of the above

Q44. Which of the following is true regarding catheter-related bacteraemia?

1. If bacteraemia is suspected, blood from the catheter tips and a minimum of two blood samples are cultured
2. When dialysis catheter-induced bacteraemia is suspected, empiric systemic intravenous antimicrobial therapy is administered
3. The best option for achieving a cure of the infection is immediate removal of the infected catheter
4. All of the above

Q45. Which of the following is true in Catheter Insertion?

1. In the early 1980s, doctors used lumen catheters, which were a rigid coaxial variety and substituted after every hemodialysis session; later, catheters were constructed from medical silicone rubber and continue to be in use till today
2. Femoral vein insertion has the biggest risk of infections
3. Fatal doses of air measuring as little as 20 mL can be aspirated in seconds through a large bore catheter
4. All of the above

Q46. Which of the following is true for sterilisation of apheresis equipments?

1. *High-pressure steam method* is used for Hemoperfusion equipments
2. *Gamma radiation method* is deployed for Cascadeflo and Plasmaflo™ (Asahi Kasei Medical)
3. *Ethylene oxide gas (EOG)* method used in sterilization can cause anaphylactoid reactions in few patients
4. All of the above

Q47. Therapeutic plasma exchange is a relatively safe procedure *but* it is contraindicated in which of the following conditions?

1. Active infection
2. Non availability of central line or large bore peripheral lines
3. ACE inhibitor treatment in last 24 hours
4. All of the above

Q48. Which of the following are *contraindications* for performing Therapeutic plasma exchange?

1. Hemodynamic instability
2. Allergy to fresh frozen plasma or albumin
3. Allergy to heparin (if heparin is the only option for anticoagulation)
4. All of the above

Q49. Which among the following is false regarding plasma exchange ?

1. Plasma exchange is usually considered a safe procedure
2. The risk of complications is 10%
3. The risk of life threatening complications is 0.025% to 4.75%
4. The vital signs are recorded every 15 minutes, allergic reactions and signs and symptoms of hypocalcaemia are monitored before, during and after the procedure

ANSWERS

Q1. Ans(1)

Q2. Ans(4)

Q3. Ans(2)

Q4. Ans(4)

Q5. Ans(4)

Q6. Ans(2)
It is added every 3 years

Q7. Ans(4)

Q8. Ans(1)

Q9. Ans(3)
The second filters are available with different pore sizes.

Q10. Ans(4)

Q11. Ans(4)

Q12. Ans(4)

Q13. Ans(4)

Q14. Ans(4)

Q15. Ans(4)

Q16. Ans(4)

Q17. Ans(4)

Q18. Ans(1)
Explanation: Peripherally implanted central catheters (PICC) are not suitable for apheresis treatments because of increased blood flows. The increase in blood flow leads to elevated pressures which may lead to PICC rupture. Temporary, short-term implantation of Central Venous Catheters (CVC) in the subclavian (SC), internal jugular (IJ), or femoral veins is permissible for apheresis. PORT (Subcutaneously implanted intravascular devices) access is positioned with catheter tunnelled into the distal superior vena cava or right atrium. High-flow dual (VORTEX) ports utilized with large-bore non-coring needles are appropriate for apheresis. Skin-tunnelled catheters (Hickman lines) are placed through jugular veins, subclavian for long-term access (exceeding 30 days).

Q19. Ans(4)
Explanation: Pinch-off syndrome (POS) is a life-threatening complication associated with implantable central venous catheters. POS is associated with infraclavicular approach of implantable catheters. The catheter should be removed immediately to avoid catheter fracture and embolization of fragments.

Q20. Ans(1)
Figure II-2. *Peripheral venous access device- short with-Infusion.* Reproduced from Michael Berry, English Wikipedia (36) Licensed under CC BY 3.0 Unported.

Figure II-3 Implanted venous access device -Port Catheter [Cropped from original photo *Recurrent breastCA.gif*] derivative by Una Smith. Public domain. Data sources: Fulcher & Frazier, 2011; Perry et al., 2018(37) licensed under a Creative Commons Attribution 4.0 International License

Q21. Ans(4)

Q22. Ans(4)

Q23. Ans(4)

Q24. Ans(4)

Q25. Ans(4)

Q26. Ans(4)

Q27. Ans(4)

Q28. Ans(4)

Q29. Ans(4)

Q30. Ans(2)

Q31. Ans(3)

Q32. Ans(3)

Q33. Ans(3)

Q34. Ans(4)

Q35. Ans(2)

Q36. Ans(4)

Q37. Ans(4)

Q38. Ans(4)
Explanation: The citrate-based anticoagulation is highly efficacious and it is used in routine exchange procedures. The unfractionated heparin (UFH) is only used as a combined therapy for paediatric apheresis. It is also used in large volume leukapheresis for adults, in membrane-based plasma exchange, LDL-apheresis, or photopheresis.

In a concomitant continuous infusion with citrate, WB:Citrate ratios are decreased to 1:25 to1:30 and heparin is bolus dosed (20-40 IU/kg). After that, continued infusion (0.1-0.5IU/kg/min) with ACT monitoring maintains clotting time to 180-210 seconds. 5000 units of heparin is added to a 500 mL ACD-A bag and infused at 1:30 WB:AC.

Q39. Ans(4)

Q40. Ans(4)

Q41. Ans(2)

Q42. Ans(4)

Q43. Ans(4)

Q44. Ans(4)

Q45. Ans(4)

Q46. Ans(4)

Q47. Ans(4)

Q48. Ans(4)

Q49. Ans(2)
Various studies have suggested the risk of complications as high as 40%

REFERENCES

1. Pham P, Schwartz J. How to approach an apheresis consultation using the American Society for Apheresis guidelines for therapeutic apheresis procedures. 2015 International Society of Blood Transfusion, ISBT Science Series. 2015;10(Suppl. 1):79–88.
2. Connelly-Smith L, Alquist CR, Aqui NA, et al. Guidelines on the use of therapeutic apheresis in clinical practice–evidence-based approach from the Writing Committee of the American Society for Apheresis: the ninth special issue. J Clin Apher. 2023;38(2):77–278
3. McLeod BC, Szczepiorkowski ZM, Weinstein R, Winters JL, editors. Apheresis: Principles and Practice. 3rd ed. Bethesda, MD: AABB Press; 2010.
4. Guyatt G, Gutterman D, Baumann MH, et al. Grading strengthof recommendations and quality of evidence in clinical guidelines: report from an American College of Chest Physicians Task Force. Chest. 2006;129:174-181.
5. Nakaji S, Yamamoto T. Membranes for therapeutic apheresis. Ther Apher [Internet].2002;6(4):267–70. Available from http://dx.doi.org/10.1046/j.1526-0968.2002.00442.x
6. Noiri E. and Hanafusa N., The Concise Manual of Apheresis Therapy. Tokyo: Springer Japan;2014
7. C. Elena Cervantes, Bloch EM, C. John Sperati. Therapeutic Plasma Exchange: Core Curriculum 2023. 2023 Feb 1;81(4):475–92.
8. Kozanoglu I *Problem Solving in Apheresis Medicine*, Switzerland: Springer Nature; 2024.
9. Jiang X, Feng J, Ye Y. Double-filtration plasmapheresis for treatment of acute renal failure in a multiple myeloma patient. Ther Apher Dial. 2014;18(3):318–9. Mineshima
10. M, Yokoi R, Horibe K, Eguchi K, Kaneko I, Agishi T, et al. Effects of operating conditions on selectivity of plasma fractionator in double filtration plasmapheresis. Ther Apher. 2001;5(6):444–8.
11. Thalgahagoda S, Webb NJ, Roberts D, Birch A, Milford DV, Tavakoli A, et al. Successful ABO incompatible renal transplantation following rituximab and DFPP after failed immunoadsorption. Pediatr Transplant. 2014;18(3):74–6.
12. Lyu R, Chen W, Hsieh S. Plasma exchange versus DFPP in the treatment of Guillain-Barre syndrome. Ther Apher Dial. 2002;6:163–6.
13. Otsubo S, Tanabe K, Shinmura H, Ishikawa N, Tokumoto T, Hattori M, et al. Effect of posttransplant double filtration plasmapheresis on recurrent focal and segmental glomerulosclerosis in renal transplant recipients. Ther Apher Dial. 2004;8(4):299–304.
14. Agishi T, Kaneko I, Hasuo Y, Sanaka T, Sudo N, Hayasaka Y, et al. DFPP utilizing new membrane technology. J Jpn Soc Dial Ther. 1981;14:61–5.
15. Hirano R, Namazuda K, Hirata N. Double filtration plasmapheresis: review of current clinical applications. Ther Apher Dial. 2021;25(2):145–51.
16. Hadid T, Hernandez M, Zeni A, Jain N. Pinch-off syndrome: a rare and serious complication of central venous catheters. BMJ Case Rep. 2020;13(1): e232417.
17. NHS Blood and Transplant. Therapeutic apheresis [Internet]. London: NHS Blood andTransplant; [cited 2026 Jan 25]. Available from: https://www.nhsbt.nhs.uk/what-we-do/diagnostic-and-therapeutic-services/therapeutic-apheresis
18. Kalantari K. The choice of vascular access for therapeutic apheresis. J Clin Apher. 2012;27:153–9.
19. Ipe TS. Vascular access for therapeutic plasma exchange. Transfusion. 2018;58(suppl 1):580–9.
20. Juric S. An innovative approach to near-infrared spectroscopy using a standard mobile device and its clinical application in the real time visualization of peripheral veins. BMC Med Inform Decis Mak. 2014;14:100.
21. Cheng JE, Hendrickson, Sidhu D, Jd MD. Therapeutic Plasma Exchange and Its Impact on Drug Levels An ACLPS Critical ReviewCaleb W. Vol. 148. MD,1,2 Christopher A. Tormey, MD,1; 2017.
22. Pham HP, DePalma H, Williams LA III. Transfusion medicine, haemostasis, apheresis review questions and case studies pretest 1. In: *Transfusion Medicine, Apheresis, and Hemostasis*. 2018. p. 2.
23. Hester JP, McCullough J, Mishler JM, Szymanski IO. Dosage regimens for citrate anticoagulants. J Clin Apher. 1983;1:149–57.
24. Weinstein R. Prevention of citrate reactions during therapeutic plasma exchange by constant infusion of calcium gluconate with the return fluid. J Clin Apher. 1996;11:204–10.
25. Bjorkman MP, Sorva AJ, Tilvis RS. Calculated serum calcium is an insufficient surrogate for measured ionized calcium. Arch Gerontol Geriatr. 2009;49(3):348–50.
26. Kim HC. Therapeutic pediatric apheresis. J Clin Apher. 2000;15(1–2):129–57.
27. Goldstein SL. Therapeutic apheresis in children: special considerations. Semin Dial.2012;25(2):165–70.
28. Sharma SK. Low Molecular Weight Heparins. Med J Armed Forces India. 1998 Jul;54(3):285-286.
29. Weitz JI. Low molecular weight heparins. N Engl J Med. 1997;338:688–698.
30. Lee G, Arepally GM. Anticoagulation techniques in apheresis: from heparin to citrate and beyond. Journal of Clinical Apheresis. 2012;27(3):117–25.
31. Arora N., *Procedures and Protocols in the Neurocritical Care Unit.* Switzerland:Springer Nature;2022.

32. Szczeklik W, Wawrzycka K, Włudarczyk A, Sega A, Nowak I, Seczyńska B, et al. Complications in patients treated with plasmapheresis in the intensive care unit. Anaesthesiol Intens Ther. 2013;45(1):7–13.
33. Holford NHG. Pharmacokinetics and pharmacodynamics: rational dosing and the timecourse of drug action. VanderahVT. Katzung BG. Basic and Clinical Pharmacology. 16th ed. New York: McGraw Hill; 2024.p.43.
34. Instructions for using Heparin as AC-Terumo BCT
35. Correia MR, Lopes CS, Barros AI, Cagigal J, Sinde J, et al. Catheter dysfunction in a child: Recognizing pinch-off syndrome. Ann Pediatr. 2025;8(1):1148.p.1.
36. Berry M. Intravenous therapy [Internet]. English Wikipedia; [cited 2026 Feb 13]. Available from: https://en.wikipedia.org/wiki/File:Intravenous_therapy.jpg. Licensed under CC BY 3.0 Unported. https://pressbooks.bccampus.ca/clinicalproceduresforsaferpatientcaretrubscn/chapter/8-3-types-of-venous-access/
37. Smith U. *Port catheter* [Internet image]. Derived from Recurrent breastCA.gif [cropped]. Public domain [cited 2026 Feb 13]. https://pressbooks.bccampus.ca/clinicalproceduresforsaferpatientcaretrubscn/chapter/8-3-types-of-venous-access/

Chapter 3

IMMUNOADSORPTION

Dr. Swapna and Dr. Priyanka

Q1. All of the following are true for processing of Plasma volume except:

1. The plasma volume exchanged is 2-2.5 Plasma volume in Immunoadsorption Plasmapheresis irrespective of body weight
2. The plasma volume exchanged is 1-1.5 Plasma volume in Double Filtration Plasmapheresis
3. The plasma volume exchanged is 1-1.5 Plasma volume in Therapeutic Plasma Exchange
4. None of the above

Q2. Which of the following is true for Immunoadsorption (IA) with respect to patient evaluation?

1. Treatment decisions with IA depends mostly on the patient's age, diagnosis, health status, complication risks, and coagulation or bleeding status
2. Immunoadsorption (IA) removes immunoglobulins mainly from plasma
3. There is no depletion of clotting factors or complement
4. All of the above

Q3. Which of the following is true regarding clearance of substances by PE, DFPP, IAPP?

1. Clearance is equal to the exchanged plasma volume in case of a simple plasma exchange
2. Clearance is less than the processed volume in double filtration plasmapheresis (DFPP)
3. Clearance is less than the processed volume in case of plasma adsorption
4. All of the above

Q4. Which of the following is true in immunoadsorption?

1. Immunoadsorption is a treatment protocol that depends on antigen–antibody interactions
2. The immunoadsorption protocol is specific to pathogenic toxins
3. The USFDA has approved two types of immunosorbents namely Immunosorba (Excorim) and Prosorba (Fresenius Hemocare)
4. All of the above

Q5. All of the following are true in removal efficiency of the adsorption process except

1. It depends on the chemical nature of the pathogens
2. The adsorbents have an upper limit for the amount of substance that can be adsorbed
3. It does not depend on the pathogen's molecular weight
4. None of the above

Q6. Which of the following is false in Immunoadsorption ?

1. The Plasma Adsorption column often processes a maximum volume of 2–3 L of plasma only
2. Plasma Adsorption is ideally not suitable for patients with a large physique because larger volume of plasma needs to be processed and it is a disadvantage
3. Some columns such as Liposorber LA-15 are reactivated and reused
4. None of the above

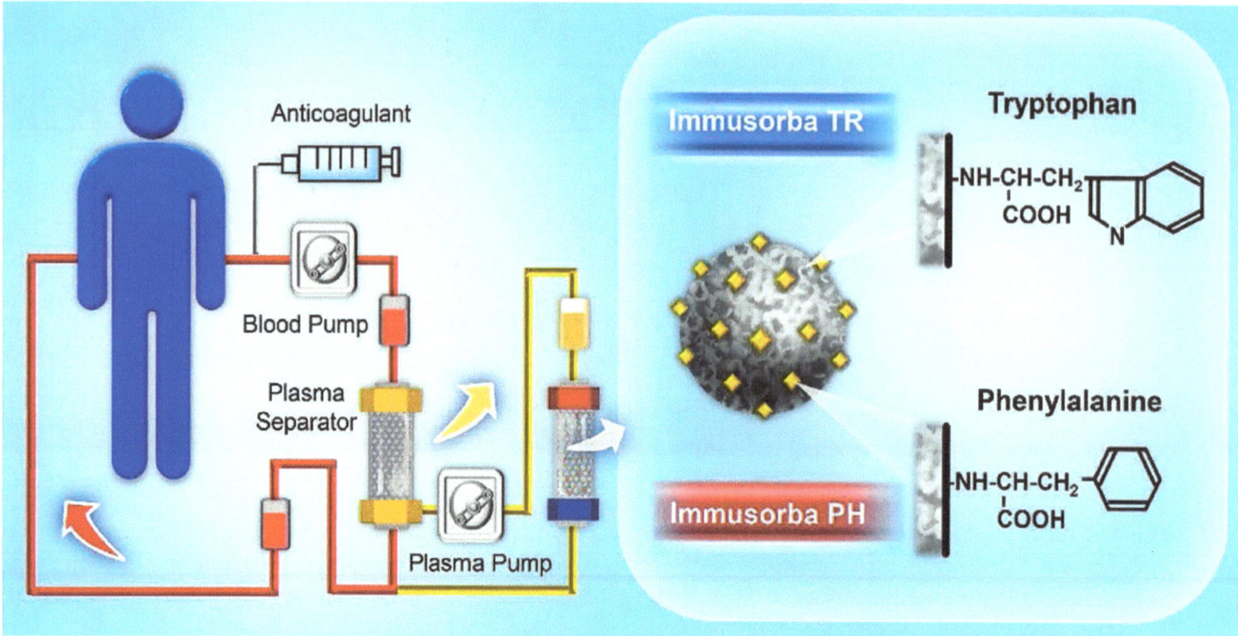

Fig III-1: A schematic illustration of immunoadsorption using Immusorba TR and Immusorba PH. Reproduced from [Yu and Ou (23) 2023 Creative Commons Attribution License (CC BY)]

Q7. The Fig III-1 is Immunoadsorption (IA), which of the following is true?

1. IA Immusorba TR is used for Autoantibodies removal
2. IA Immusorba PH is used for Immune complexes removal
3. Both of the above
4. None of the above

Q8. All of the following are true in Immunoadsorption with respect to Liposorber and Selesorb except

1. Liposorber and Selesorb use the same ligand (*dextran sulfate*), but have different pore sizes
2. Liposorber and Selesorb use different ligands, but have same pore sizes
3. In the adsorptive method fluid is not removed and hence fluid *supplementation is not* necessary
4. Selesorb adsorbs *immune complexes and antibodies*, while, Liposorber adsorbs the larger *low-density lipoprotein molecule*

Q9. All of the following are true in the mechanisms of Immunoadsorption except

1. The adsorptive devices are divided into two groups depending on the adsorption mechanism used (eg *hydrophobic or electrostatic* interaction)
2. Each type of plasma adsorption column has a *different* maximum adsorption capacity
3. Immusorba PH-350 column has phenylalanine as a ligand that selectively adsorbs via *electrostatic* interactions and eliminates anti-DNA antibodies and rheumatoid factors
4. None of the above

Q10. Which of the following is true in Selective plasmapheresis?

1. ImmunoAdsorption (IA), Plasma Adsorption Perfusion (PAP), Lipoprotein Apheresis (LA) are all types of selective plasmapheresis
2. The plasma volume (that needs to be treated) is directed into a column where the selective adsorption happens and the pathogens are eliminated
3. The same purified plasma (once the adsorption is completed) is returned to the patient
4. All of the above

Q11. Adsorption using ion exchange resin was performed for a patient suffering hepatic encephalopathy for the first time

1. by Scechter in 1958
2. by Scechter in 1950
3. by Cohn in 1950
4. by Cohn in 1958

Q12. Which of the following is false for the Immunoadsorption columns?

1. Liposorber (LA-40S, LA-15) columns can eliminate LDL selectively with a large bore diameter
2. Selesorb can eliminate immune complexes, anti-DNA antibodies, and anti-cardiolipin antibodies better with a small -bore diameter
3. Columns using dextran sulfate as a ligand selectively eliminate substances through electrostatic interactions between the negative and positive charges of dextran sulfate
4. None of the above

Q13. All of the following are true in the features of Immunoadsorption (IA) except

1. IA is employed in *different autoimmune diseases* to remove immunoglobulins, immune complexes, and circulating anti bodies
2. The loss of immunoglobulins is not accompanied with that of electrolytes or plasma proteins
3. *Citrate is used* in combination with *heparin* for anticoagulation
4. None of the above

Q14. All of the following are true regarding IA Therasorb devices except

1. Ig-Therasorb® (Miltenyi Biotec, Bergisch Gladbach, Germany): Each adsorber column contains 150 mL Sepharose
2. Therasorb is coupled with polyclonal sheep antibodies to capture both heavy as well as light chains human IgG
3. The immunoglobulin-binding capacity is approximately 4.0 g
4. None of the above

Q15. All of the following are true regarding IgG absorption and adsorbents except

1. Immunosorba® and Ligasorb® (Fresenius Medical Care, Bad Homburg, Germany): use Reusable protein A-based adsorber columns
2. The IgG subclasses 1,2,4 are removed
3. The removal rate of IgG-3, is noticeable only when high plasma volumes are processed
4. None of the above

Q16. Which of the following are true regarding IgG elimination?

1. All the subtypes of IgG are removed with Double Filtration Plasmapheresis
2. Plasma Adsorption cannot remove all subtypes of IgG
3. Plasma Adsorption with a tryptophan-conjugated column can adsorb IgG 3 but not IgG 4
4. All of the above

Q17. All of the following are true regarding Immunoadsorption (IA) indications according to ASFA guidelines except

1. IA is a therapeutic method for rapid elimination of persisting iso hemagglutinins in patients with PRCA after ABO-I HCT
2. IA is the treatment of choice for removal of coagulation factor inhibitors (both allo and auto inhibitors)
3. IA is the therapeutic method for Refractory Immune thrombocytopenia, Cryoglobulinemia, Paraneoplastic neurological syndrome
4. None of the above

Q18. Which of the following are types of adsorption columns?

1. Carbon adsorption
2. PMX-DHP
3. Beta 2 micro globulin
4. All of the above

Q19. Blood Adsorption Methods for endotoxins includes:

1. A polymyxin-B-immobilized fiber column (PMX cartridge, Toraymyxin™) acts via electrostatic adsorption between lipid A and cationic amino acid in polymyxin-B
2. A polymyxin-B-immobilized fiber column (PMX cartridge, Toraymyxin™) acts via hydrophobic adsorption between the fatty acid moiety in lipid A and the linear structure of methyl octanoic acid in polymyxin-B for endotoxin absorbtion
3. They are used for infections caused by Gram Negative Rods
4. All of the above

Q20. All of the following are true regarding the removal of Bilirubin and Bile acid except
1. Columns to adsorb bilirubin and bile acid are Plasorba BRS-350 and Medisorba BL-300
2. These columns use a styrene-divinyl benzene copolymer, an ion exchange resin
3. The ligand selectively eliminates negatively charged bilirubin and bile acid
4. None of the above

Q21. Which of the following is true for Plasorba Column usage?
1. Plasorba BRS-350 Columns are indicated to adsorb bilirubin when level is greater than 30 mg/dL
2. There is no need for replacement of plasma during the procedure
3. It is used to treat patients suffering from protein allergy
4. All of the above

Q22. All of the following are true in IA with Lixelle except
1. The Lixelle is used for removal of Beta2- macroglobulin
2. The Lixelle device is often recommended along with hemodialysis for patients affected with secondary amyloidosis undergoing long term hemodialysis
3. The Lixelle device uses Hexadecyl-group ligands on porous cellulose beads with a 460 nm pore size
4. None of the above

Q23. Which of the following is true in Activated Charcoal?
1. The Activated Charcoal is not a biocompatible material
2. Chemical adsorption is performed with activated charcoal
3. The *encapsulation feature* facilitates adsorption from whole blood without causing platelet activation or haemolysis
4. All of the above

Q24. Which of the following is true for Hemosorba type of adsorption?
1. It uses activated charcoal and the micropores that can trap chemical materials reversibly at 500 - 1,000 kDa
2. The mode of action is hydrophobic adsorption
3. It is indicated for treating poisoning from toxins like agrichemicals, drugs such as sleeping pills, and anti-arrhythmic drugs
4. All of the above

Q25. Which of the following is true regarding apheresis in COVID-19?
1. Immunoadsorption was used in critically ill COVID-19 patients with uncontrolled cytokine release
2. Immunoadsorption using Therasorb–Ig flex connected to a LIFE-21 plasmapheresis platform was used in Covid-19 for convalescent plasma donation
3. Selective C-Reactive Protein apheresis was proposed as a method to reduce its levels in COVID-19 patients
4. All of the above

Q26. Which of the following is false in selective IA?
1. Selective IA removes antibodies directed towards a specific antigen; was pioneered in Sweden
2. Selective IA, worked effectively in ABO-incompatible organ transplantation (If anti-A and anti-B have to be removed, two columns are placed in series)
3. One single-use column selectively removes over 90% of the target antibodies in case of ABO-incompatible organ transplantation
4. None of the above

Q27. The indications for Molecular Adsorbent Recirculating System (MARS) include which of the following?
1. A transplant candidate suffering from acute fulminant liver failure
2. When a listed transplant candidate is suffering from acute on chronic liver failure
3. MARS is used as a bridge to recovery or as a bridge to transplant
4. All of the above

Q28. Identify the device/circuit in the Fig III-2 that was used since 1990s

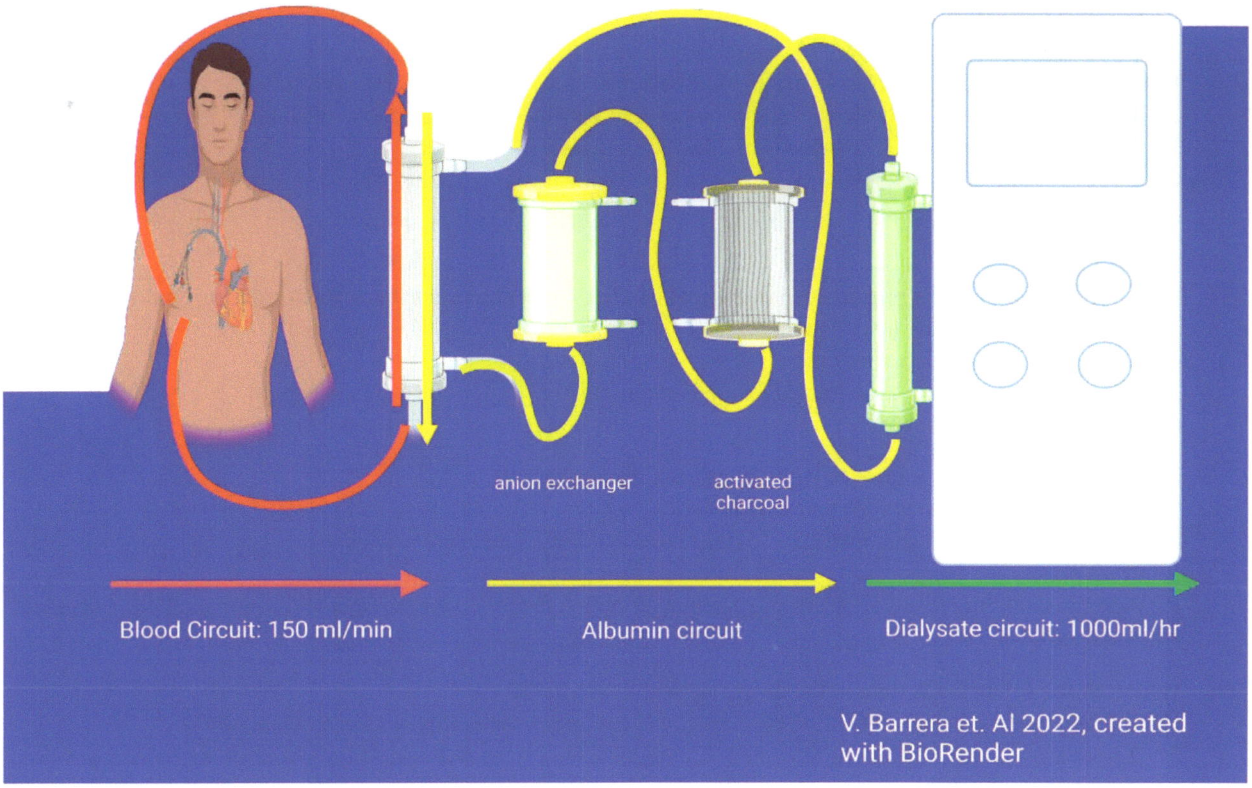

Fig III-2: Adapted from Villanueva et al. (27) 2023 CCBY (4.0) (Description in answer key)

1. MARS (Molecular Adsorbent Recirculating System)
2. Prometheus
2. SPAD (Single pass albumin dialysis)
4. None of the above

Q29. Molecular adsorbent recirculating system (MARS) is an extracorporeal hepatic support system that works on the mechanisms of

1. Dialysis
2. Ultrafiltration
3. Adsorption
4. All of the above

Q30. The following in MARS (Molecular Adsorbent Recirculating System) is true

1. MARS is a relatively recently reported blood purification method and is costly
2. The main mechanism involves separating albumin binding substances from the blood and the water-soluble substances are removed by the bicarbonate dialysis fluid
3. Albumin binding substances are adsorbed by the activated carbon as well as ion-exchange resin and this purified albumin floating fluid is reused
4. All of the above

Q31. The FDA has approved the use of MARS Molecular Adsorbent Recirculating System for Hepatic Encaphalopathy improvement in patients with

1. Chronic liver disease
2. Acute Liver Failure
3. Chronic Kidney Failure
4. All of the above

Q32. MARS Molecular Adsorbent Recirculating System) is relatively contraindicated if there is

1. An increased risk of coagulopathy (example: disseminated intravascular coagulation)
2. Uncontrolled sepsis
3. Uncontrolled hemorrhage
4. All of the above

Q33. Which of the following are true in usage of MARS Molecular Adsorbent Recirculating System)?

1. There is no increase in citrate concentration (as seen with other extra corporeal techniques Plasma Diafiltration, Plasma Exchange with Continuous Hemo Dia Filtration)
2. Bilirubin removal is moderate
3. Fibrinogen retention is good
4. All of the above

Q34. Which of the following is applicable in usage of MARS Molecular Adsorbent Recirculating System)?

1. It negatively influences coagulation
2. It also increases prothrombin time
3. It may also alter coagulation-related factors such as factor V
4. All of the above

Q35. Which of the following is false in Hemoperfusion devices?

1. Prometheus uses plasma filtration with help of adsorption columns and leads to platelets reduction
2. MARS uses activated charcoal/anionic substances, cholestyramine, anion exchange resin, and has the advantage of nil platelets reduction
3. Adsorba uses drug removal by means of activated carbon particles and is associated with reduction in platelets
4. None of the above

Q36. Which of the following is true in leukocyte apheresis (LCAP)?

1. The leukocyte apheresis (LCAP) Cellsorba-EX™ device uses non-woven fabric technology
2. It used a polyester ultra-micro fibre of 1–3 mm diameter for the removal of lymphoid cells, granulocytes, and monocytes
3. The target processing volume is 2 L
4. All of the above

Q37. Which of the following regarding LCAP in Rheumatoid arthritis is false?

1. Rheumatoid arthritis is treated with pulse LCAP using a bigger column (CS-180S)
2. This column can process a greater volume of blood (5 L or 100 mL/kg)
3. Pulse LCAP is more effective for treatment of rheumatoid arthritis compared with conventional low volume (3 L) treatment using the CS-100
4. None of the above

Q38. Which of the following is true in GCAP?

1. The Adacolumn™ device, using granulocyte apheresis (GCAP), has bio incompatible beads
2. There is activation of complement 3b (C3b)
3. The activated C3b binds to the surface of the beads and induces C3b-dependent chemotaxis to granulocytes and monocytcs, but not to lymphocytes
4. All of the above

Q39. Which of the following is true for GCAP Granulocyte Cytapheresis?

1. About 1.5-2.0 litres of Blood volume is treated
2. Cellulose acetate is the adsorbent and eliminates 30–50% of granulocytes and monocytes
3. The efficacy of GCAP is proved for the treatment of Crohn's disease and Ulcerative Colitis
4. All of the above

Q40. A serious adverse effect reported with the use of several immunoadsorption columns, including the Protein A Silica (PAS) column and the Dextran Sulfate (SDS) system, involves which class of medications?

1. β-blockers, causing severe bradycardia and hypotension
2. Angiotensin-converting enzyme (ACE) inhibitors, leading to severe hypotensive reactions
3. High-dose corticosteroids, causing electrolyte disturbances
4. Nonsteroidal anti-inflammatory drugs (NSAIDs), causing acute renal failure

Q41. The Immunosorba column, which uses Protein A Agarose (PAA), is characterized by regenerative capacity. The capacity for continuous, long-term use is enabled by which principle of operation?

1. The column binding sites regenerate naturally over time during treatment, allowing continuous flow without interruption
2. The plasma is treated in batches that are eluted with an acidic solution, restoring the column's binding capacity for subsequent use
3. Two columns are used in parallel; when one is saturated, plasma flow is switched to the second column while the first is regenerated with an acidic fluid and buffer
4. PAA columns employ a filtration principle that allows the pathogenic substances to pass through to waste while retaining the larger, beneficial plasma constituents

Q42. The first clinical report for LDL apheresis detailed two cases of familial hypercholesterolemia in

1. 1975
2. 1980
3. 1982
4. 1990

Q43. Which of the following is true in LDL apheresis?

1. Liposorber systems (Kaneka) and double filtration plasmapheresis (DFPP) systems are used
2. Removal rates are similar between the two systems
3. LDL reduction achieved is by 50-70%
4. All of the above

Q44. Low density lipoprotein (LDL), is recognized as a causative molecule of atherosclerosis

1. With a specific gravity of 1.019–1.063 g/mL and a particle size of 19–22 nm
2. With a specific gravity of 1.029–1.063 g/mL and a particle size of 18–19 nm
3. With a specific gravity of 1.009–1.003 g/mL and a particle size of 19–22 nm
4. With a specific gravity of 1.019–1.063 g/mL and a particle size of 23–29 nm

Q45. Indications for LDL apheresis include

1. Familial hypercholesterolemia (FH)
2. Peripheral arterial disease (PAD) of lower extremities
3. Focal segmental glomerulosclerosis (FSGS)
4. All of the above

Q46. Persistent cases of Familial hypercholesterolemia (FH) are taken up for LDL apheresis when

1. Hypercholesterolemia (total cholesterol ≥ 220 mg/dL or LDL cholesterol ≥ 140 mg/dL) refractory to drug administration
2. Hypercholesterolemia (total cholesterol ≥ 250 mg/dL or LDL cholesterol ≥ 200 mg/dL) refractory to drug administration
3. Hypercholesterolemia (total cholesterol ≥ 220 mg/dL or LDL cholesterol ≥ 140 mg/dL) responding to drug administration
4. Hypercholesterolemia (total cholesterol ≥ 260 mg/dL or LDL cholesterol ≥ 140 mg/dL) refractory to drug administration

Q47. ACE inhibitor administration should be discontinued prior to LDL Apheresis by at least

1. 4-5 days
2. 2-3 days
3. 6-7 days
4. 10 days

Q48. ACE inhibitor administration should be discontinued prior to LDL Apheresis to avoid

1. Anaphylactoid Reactions
2. Hyperbilirubinemia
3. Hypernatremia
4. Hypermagnesimia

Q49. Precautions taken for LDL Apheresis includes all except

1. Screening for gastrointestinal bleeding before LDL apheresis
2. Monitoring fibrinogen levels during the duration of treatment
3. Monitoring magnesium levels during the duration of treatment
4. Assessing the necessity of lowering the dose of antiplatelet drugs or prostaglandin analogues

Q50. LDL apheresis is indicated in FSGS when Nephrotic syndrome

1. Has total cholesterol more than 250 mg/dL
2. Is resistant to corticosteroid therapy
3. Has total cholesterol ≥ 220 mg/dL or LDL cholesterol ≥ 180 mg/dL)
4. 1 and 2

Q51. LDL apheresis involves all except

1. Total plasma volume treated is usually 3–5 L/session
2. Removal of positively charged particles as well as low density lipoprotein cholesterol
3. Promotion of bleeding tendencies because of the adsorption of endogenous coagulation factors
4. Removal of negatively charged particles as well as low density lipoprotein cholesterol

Q52. Typically, LDL Apheresis is indicated in the following types of Familial hypercholesterolemia

1. Homozygous and heterozygous FH unresponsive to conventional drug therapies, especially if homozygous FH with LDL cholesterol levels >500 mg/dL
2. Heterozygous FH with LDL cholesterol levels >300 mg/dL or heterozygous FH with high risk of cardiovascular disease and LDL cholesterol >200 mg/dL
3. Heterozygous FH with cardiovascular disease diabetes and LDL cholesterol >160 mg/dL
4. All of the above

Q53. Which of the following is false regarding the adsorbents used?

1. Cytokines are adsorbed by Hydrophobic resin after plasma filtration in CPFA (coupled plasma filtration adsorption device; Bellco, Mirandola, Italy) and it is currently available in Europe
2. In Prosorba (Fresenius Medical Care, Bad Homburg, Germany);Silica-Protein A absorbs IgG IgA IgM; is used in treatment of FSGS, Henoch-Schönlein, vasculitis, SLE, Rheumatoid Arthritis
3. Plasmapheresis derived plasma exposed to Sepharose-CL beads-peptide ligands in *Globaffin* (Fresenius-Affina Medical Care, Bad Homburg, Germany); absorbs IgG, IgA, IgM, and is used for treatment of RA, SLE, Transplant rejection, Goodpasture syndrome
4. None of the above

ANSWERS

Q1. Ans(4)	Q2. Ans(4)	Q3. Ans(4)	Q4. Ans(4)	Q5. Ans(4)	Q6. Ans(4)
Q7. Ans(3)	Q8. Ans(2)	Q9. Ans(3)	Q10. Ans(4)	Q11. Ans(1)	Q12. Ans(4)
Q13. Ans(4)	Q14. Ans(4)	Q15. Ans(4)	Q16. Ans(4)	Q17. Ans(4)	Q18. Ans(4)
Q19. Ans(4)	Q20. Ans(4)	Q21. Ans(4)	Q22. Ans(4)	Q23. Ans(4)	Q24. Ans(4)
Q25. Ans(4)	Q26. Ans(4)	Q27. Ans(4)	Q28. Ans(1)	Q29. Ans(4)	Q30. Ans(4)
Q31. Ans(1)	Q32. Ans(4)	Q33. Ans(4)	Q34. Ans(4)	Q35. Ans(4)	Q36. Ans(4)
Q37. Ans(4)	Q38. Ans(4)	Q39. Ans(4)	Q40. Ans(2)	Q41. Ans(3)	Q42. Ans(1)
Q43. Ans(4)	Q44. Ans(1)	Q45. Ans(4)	Q46. Ans(1)	Q47. Ans(2)	Q48. Ans(1)
Q49. Ans(3)	Q50. Ans(4)	Q51. Ans(4)	Q52. Ans(4)	Q53. Ans(4)	

REFERENCES

1. Kozanoğlu I. *Problem Solving in Apheresis Medicine*. Switzerland:Springer Nature;2024.
2. Hanafusa N. Theoretical basis of pathogenic substance removal during plasmapheresis. Ther Apher Dial 2011;15(5):421–430
3. Abutalib SA, Padmanabhan A, Pham HP, Worel N, editors. Best practices of apheresis in hematopoietic cell transplantation. 2020th ed. Cham, Switzerland: Springer International Publishing; 2019.
4. Altobelli C, Anastasio P, Cerrone A, Signoriello E, Lus G, Pluvio C, et al. Therapeutic plasmapheresis: A revision of literature. Kidney Blood Press Res [Internet]. 2023;48(1):66–78. Available from: http://dx.doi.org/10.1159/000528556
5. Süfke S, Lehnert H, Uhlenbusch-Körwer I, GebauerF., Safety aspects of immunoadsorption in IgG removal using a single-use, multiple-pass protein a immunoadsorber (LIGASORB): clinical investigation in healthy volunteers. Ther Apher Dial 2017; 21(4):405–413
6. Koefoed-Nielsen P, Bistrup C, Christiansen M. Protein a immunoadsorption may hamper the decision to transplant due to interference with CDC crossmatch results. J Clin Apher 2017;32(3):163–169
7. Tseke P, Griveas I. Immunoadsorption and covid 19 pandemic. Transfus Apher Sci. 2022; 61(6):103599.
8. Singh A. K. *Core Concepts in Dialysis and Continuous Therapies*. Switzerland:Springer:2016
9. Mitzner SR. Extracorporeal liver support-albumin dialysis with the Molecular Adsorbent Recirculating System (MARS). Ann Hepatol. 2011 May;10 Suppl 1:S21-8.
10. Mielnicki W, Dyla A, Karczewski M. Clinical effectiveness of MARS treatment - multidirectional analysis of positive clinical response to treatment. Clin Exp Hepatol. 2019 Nov;5(4):271-278.
11. Noiri E. and Hanafusa N., The Concise Manual of Apheresis Therapy. Tokyo;Japan: Springer; 2014
12. Pőcze, B., Fazakas, J., Zádori, G., Görög, D., Kóbori, L., Dabasi, E., Mándli, T., Piros, L., Smudla, A., Szabó, T., Toronyi, É., Tóth, S., Tőzsér, G., Végső, G., Doros, A., & Nemes, B.MARS therapy, the bridging to liver retransplantation – Three cases from the Hungarian liver transplant program. *Interventional Medicine & Applied Science*, 2013; *5*(2), 70.
13. Gerth HU, Pohlen M, Thölking G, Pavenstädt H, Brand M, Hüsing-Kabar A, et al. Molecular adsorbent recirculating system can reduce short-term mortality among patients with acute-on-Chronic Liver Failure-A retrospective analysis. Crit Care Med [Internet]. 2017;45(10):1616–24.
14. Mitzner SR, Stange J, Klammt S, Risler T, Erley CM, Bader BD, Berger ED, Lauchart W, Peszynski P, Freytag J, Hickstein H, Loock J, Löhr JM, Liebe S, Emmrich J, Korten G, Schmidt R. Improvement of hepatorenal syndrome with extracorporeal albumin dialysis MARS: results of a prospective, randomized, controlled clinical trial. Liver Transpl. 2000; 6(3):277-86.
15. Jalan R, Sen S, Williams R. Prospects for extracorporeal liver support. Gut. 2004 Jun;53(6):890-8.
16. Yoo SW, Ki MJ, Kim D, Kim SK, Park S, Han HJ, Lee HB. Bleeding complications associated with the molecular adsorbent recirculating system: a retrospective study. Acute Crit Care. 2021;36(4):322-331.
17. McLeod BC, Szczepiorkowski ZM, Weinstein R, Winters JL, editors. Apheresis: Principles and Practice. 3rd ed. Bethesda, MD: AABB; 2010.
18. Thompson GR, Lowenthal R, Myant NB Plasma exchange in the management of homozygous familial hypercholesterolaemia. Lancet 1975; 1:1208–11
19. Feingold KR, Grunfeld C. Lipoprotein apheresis. In: Feingold KR, Anawalt B, Boyce A, etal., editors. Endotext South Dartmouth (Ma).MDText.com, Inc January; 2020.p 18.
20. Rönspeck W, Brinckmann R, Egner R, Gebauer F, Winkler D, Jekow P, Wallukat G, Müller J, Kunze R. Peptide based adsorbers for therapeutic immunoadsorption. Ther Apher Dial. 2003;7:91–7
21. Hidaka T, Suzuki K, Matsuki Y, Takamizawa-Matsumoto M, Kataharada K, IshizukaT, et al. Evaluation of adsorption selectivity dextran sulfate bound cellulose beads for the removal of anti-DNA antibodies. Ther Apher. 1999;3(1):75–80
22. Guan M, Wang H, Wang F, Liang S, Ling L, Wang B, Zhang L. Lipoprotein apheresis: an established therapeutic modality for homozygous familial hypercholesterolemia patients refractory to PCSK9 inhibitors: a case report and literature review. Thromb J. 2024; 22(1):85.
23. Yu, Y., & Ou, L. The development of immunosorbents for the treatment of systemic lupus erythematosus via hemoperfusion. *Frontiers in Medicine*, 2023;*9*, 1035150.p.4.
24. Mitzner, Steffen R. "Extracorporeal liver support-albumin dialysis with the Molecular Adsorbent Recirculating System (MARS)." *Annals of hepatology* 10.S1 (2016): 21-28. https://www-ncbi-nlm-nih-gov.proxy-hs.researchport.umd.edu/pubmed/21566251
25. Hanish, Steven I., et al. "Molecular adsorbent recirculating system effectively replaces hepatic function in severe acute liver failure." *Annals of surgery* 266.4 (2017): 677-684. https://www.ncbi.nlm.nih.gov/pubmed/28692474
26. He, Guo-Lin, et al. "Meta-analysis of survival with the molecular adsorbent recirculating system for liver failure." *International journal of clinical and experimental medicine* 8.10 (2015): 17046. https://www.ncbi.nlm.nih.gov/pubmed/26770295

27. Villanueva VB, Barrera Amoro´ s DA, Castillo Echeverria EI, Budar-Ferna´ ndez LF, Salas Nolasco OI, Juncos LA and Rizo-Topete L. Extracorporeal blood purification inpatients with liver failure: Considerations for the low-and-middle income countries of Latin America. Front. Nephrol. 2023;3:938710.p.6.

28. Braun N, Gutenberger S, Erley CM, Risler T. Immunoglobulin and circulating immune complex kinetics during immunoadsorption onto protein A sepharose. Trans Sci. (1997) 19:25–31. 10.1016/S0955-3886(97)00099-4

29. Samuelsson G. What's happening? Protein A columns: current concepts, and recent advances. Trans Sci. (1999) 21:215–7. 10.1016/S0955-3886(99)00096-X

Chapter 4

DOUBLE FILTRATION PLASMAPHERESIS (DFPP)

Dr. Swapna and Dr. Priyanka

Q1. Which among the following is true regarding DFPP apheresis instruments?
1. The filtration devices necessary for DFPP are not licensed in the United States
2. The filtration devices are available in Europe, Canada, and Asia
3. DFPP is given increased importance in the ninth edition of the ASFA Guidelines
4. All of the above

Q2. In Double filtration Plasmapheresis (DFPP) all of the following are true except
1. DFPP is designed to selectively remove immunoglobulins (IgA, IgM, IgD, and IgE) from the plasma
2. IgG is the most commonly targeted immunoglobulin and 80% IgG elimination efficiency can be achieved
3. Evaflux 2A ® or Cascade flo EC-20W ® are plasma component separators
4. None of the above

Q3. All of the following are true in DFPP fluid supplementation except
1. Albumin is commonly used as replacement fluid with DFPP
2. The volume of replacement fluid equals the volume discarded by the plasma component separator
3. Fluid supplementation is needed when DFPP method is used for removal of high-molecular-weight substances such as LDL or hepatitis C virus
4. DFPP requires less fluid supplementation compared to that of Plasma Exchange

Q4. All of the following are true regarding *replacement* in DFPP except
1. The volume of waste fluid is small
2. Waste fluid contains large amounts of high oncotic pressure substances
3. FFP cannot be used for fluid supplementation because of its lower oncotic pressure
4. None of the above

Q5. Which of the following is *false* regarding replacement in DFPP?
1. The serum albumin levels and haematocrit values of the patient determine the volume of replacement fluid
2. Immunoglobulins cannot be replenished as FFP is not the fluid of choice for replacement
3. Coagulation factors cannot be replenished as FFP is not the fluid of choice for replacement
4. None of the above

Q6. Which of the following is true in DFPP *membranes*?
1. All membrane plasma separators and plasma component fractionators have hollow fibre membranes and have resemblance to haemodialysis
2. The techniques of DFFP and Haemodialysis are different as membrane pore sizes are different
3. The pore size of a *membrane plasma separator* differs by 0.1 mm, and that of a *plasma component fractionator* used to separate albumin and globulin differs by 0.01 mm
4. All of the above

Q7. Which of the following is false in the DFPP *process*?
1. The quantity of pathogenic substance in plasma needs to be evaluated before selecting the plasma separator (DFPP)
2. The second plasma filtration step of DFPP aims to separate useful substances (albumin) from high molecular weight pathogenic substances
3. The advantage of DFPP includes return of useful substances
4. None of the above

Q8. The targeted substances are removed by therapeutic apheresis procedures with respect to decreasing specificity by the following order

1. Plasma Adsorption, DFPP, Plasma Exchange
2. Plasma Exchange, Plasma Adsorption, DFPP
3. DFPP, Plasma Adsorption, Plasma Exchange
4. DFPP, Plasma Exchange, Plasma Adsorption

Q9. DFFP is used for the removal of which of the following?

1. M proteins
2. Toxins or wastes excreted by the liver
3. Hepatitis C virus, hepatitis B virus, HIV, Corona virus
4. All of the above

Q10. Which of the following is false during the double filtration plasmapheresis (DFPP) procedure?

1. Oncotic pressure changes are monitored with the help of a *Crit-Line In-Line Monitor*™ [In-Line Diagnostics, Kaysville, UT] (Fresenius Medical Care AG & Co. KGaA, Bad Homburg, Germany)
2. The blood volume ideally should not *decrease beyond 10%*
3. When blood volume changes greatly, the *albumin infusion rate* is increased
4. None of the above

Q11. Which of the following are true regarding sieving coefficient for DFPP?

1. The amount of target substance returned depends on the sieving coefficient (SC) of the second filter
2. The SC is calculated as the concentration of the filtrate (Cf) divided by the concentration at the filter inlet (Ci) (SC = Cf/Ci)
3. DFPP clearance corresponds to the processed plasma volume multiplied by 1 minus the SC (1 − SC)
4. All of the above

Q12. Which of the following is true in DFPP Clearance?

1. For a substance with an SC of 0.4, the processed plasma volume is multiplied by 1 minus 0.4, or 0.6 (processed plasma volume × 0.6 = DFPP clearance)
2. Thus, a processed plasma volume of 1.4 plasma volume results in a DFPP clearance of 43.1% of the pretreatment value ($e^{-(1.4 \times 0.6)}$) = 0.431)
3. The SC of a substance that is small enough to pass through the filter is 1and the SC of a substance that is bigger than the pore size and cannot be filtered at all is 0
4. All of the above

Q13. Which of the following is true for DFPP regarding IgG removal?

1. The second filter used cannot remove the pathogenic substances completely and some portion returns to the circulation
2. The level of IgG usually decreases by 50% after each treatment, and it depends on the pathologic condition
3. If three DFPP treatments are performed every other day, the IgG level will fall to about one-eighth of baseline level provided the production rate is not high
4. All of the above

Q14. Which of the following is true regarding the sizes of the Plasma fractionators (second filter) used?

1. When Lipoproteins are the target,(molecular weight of 2,400,000 Da.) the plasma fractionator (EC-**50W**) with the largest pore size and number of pores is used
2. When IgG is the target, (the molecular weight of IgG is 200,000–300,000 Da.) the EC-**20W** plasma fractionator is used
3. When IgM is the target (molecular weight of 950,000 Da,) the EC-**40W** fractionator is used
4. All of the above

Q15. All the mechanisms are true in Plasma diafiltration (PDF) except:

1. Plasma diafiltration (PDF) is a blood purification therapy where simple plasma exchange (PE) is performed with a *selective* membrane plasma separator having a sieving coefficient 0.3 for albumin
2. PDF is a simpler method when compared to plasma exchange with continuous hemodiafiltration (CHDF) and uses only one plasma separator
3. PDF can remove both water-soluble and albumin bound substances
4. None of the above

Q16. Plasma Diafiltration is useful for patients with

1. Acute liver failure
2. Severe sepsis
3. Acute pancreatitis
4. All of the above

Q17. Which of the following is false during the performance of Plasma diafiltration?

1. Dialysis is also performed during this type of selective plasma filtration
2. The membrane has a sieving coefficient of 0 for fibrinogen and immunoglobulin M
3. PDF is useful for patients with intoxication
4. None of the above

Q18. In Plasma diafiltration (PDF), which of the following technical and clinical *feature* is false?

1. The Evacure EC-2A plasma separator with a pore size of 0.01 mm, smaller than that of conventional plasma separation membranes (0.2–0.4 mm) is used
2. The membrane can *selectively remove low and intermediate molecular weight* albumin bound substances and does not retain high molecular weight proteins such as fibrinogen and immunoglobulin M
3. PDF is performed for 24 h continuously, and it depends on the patient's condition
4. PDF is performed with a 5% albumin solution instead of FFP when there is absence of disseminated intravascular coagulation (DIC) or bleeding tendency

Q19. While applying the Plasma diafiltration (PDF), the following is true

1. The dialysate flows outside the plasma separator
2. Continuous Haemodialysis is performed using a PDF circuit
3. PDF is performed for 8h once a day as a single session
4. All of the above

Q20. Compared with haemodialysis, In DFPP thermo mode

1. There is a longer circuit configuration since there are two modules (a plasma side circuit and a blood side circuit)
2. The priming volume is approximately 400 mL and more
3. Hypoalbuminemia occurs due to the lower recovery rate of albumin in a plasma component membrane
4. All of the above

Q21. In Double Filtration Plasmapheresis Thermo-Mode (DF Thermo), the following is true in the mechanism:

1. DF thermo is a type of double filtration plasmapheresis (DFPP) where there is no requirement for fluid replacement when a large pore size *plasma component membrane* is used
2. With DF thermo, warming the plasma to 108 °F maintains the performance of plasma frac tionation
3. Heating increases the plasma processing volume and either maintains or improves the sieving coefficient
4. All of the above

Q22. In Double Filtration Plasmapheresis Thermo-Mode (DF Thermo), the following is true with respect to removal:

1. DF thermo often is used to remove the IgM fraction
2. DF thermo often is used to remove the LDL fraction
3. DF thermo often is used to remove viruses with a higher molecular weight
4. All of the above

Q23. In Double Filtration Plasmapheresis Thermo-Mode (DF Thermo), the following is true for indications and features:

1. It is used in Patients with HCV genotype II (1b) when serum RNA level >100 KIU/mL immediately after interferon therapy
2. DF thermo requires the use of three pumps: a blood pump, a plasma separation pump, and a recirculation pump
3. The KM-9000, KPS-8800Ce (Kawasumi Laboratories Inc.) is used for DF thermo
4. All of the above

Q24. Double Filtration Plasmapheresis Thermo-Mode (DF Thermo) is used in the following indications:

1. Macroglobulinemia (sequential treatments once a week for 3 months)
2. Focal segmental glomerulosclerosis when patients do not respond with conventional treatment
3. Focal segmental glomerulosclerosis when patients present with nephrotic status, and serum cholesterol level >250 mg/dL
4. All of the above

Q25. Which of the following is true in cryofiltration?

1. The cryofiltration method indicates *exposure of plasma to 37°C* and *room temperatures 25°C* and avoiding freezing
2. One approach eliminates *cryoproteins*, specifically cryoglobulins that precipitate at 4°C. The filter AP06M (Asahi Medical, Tokyo, Japan) is commonly used
3. The other method of cryofiltration eliminates *cryogel* and *cold insoluble proteins* with a heparin core, at temperatures ranging from 2 to 10°C. The AP06M, the AC1740 (Asahi Medical) filters along with the Evaflux-4A (Kuraray Company, Osaka, Japan) are used
4. All of the above

Q26. All of the following are true in Cryofiltration except:

1. Cryofiltration is a modification of double filtration plasmapheresis (DFPP) that involves cooling pathogenic proteins in the separated plasma
2. Cryofiltration is based on the formation of cryoglobulin or cryogel
3. Cryogel is an agglutination complex comprising fibrinogen, fibronectin, fibrin split products
4. None of the above

Q27. Cryofiltration circuit includes the following in the circuit:

1. Cooling system and warming device
2. Secondary membrane pressure monitoring
3. Line for washing secondary membrane
4. All of the above

Q28. Cryofiltration is used to treat patients with cryoglobulinemia and which of the following is true?

1. Cryoglobulin is the collective term for *abnormal proteins* [(including single immunoglobulins and multi-immunoglobulins (mainly IgG or IgM), that clump into a gel at 39.2 °F and dissolve at 98.6 °F]
2. Indications include *essential cryoglobulinemia or secondary cryoglobulinemia* (seen in macroglobulinemia, multiple myeloma, connective tissue disease, and hepatitis C infection)
3. EC-50W/Eva flux 5A is used as *second membrane*
4. All of the above

Q29. In cryofiltration, the following is true regarding the replacement

1. Replacement fluid generally is not required
2. Replacement of albumin is considered during multiple washings of the secondary membrane to correct hypoalbuminemia
3. If severe clotting factor deficiency occurs due to multiple washings of the secondary membrane, either the replacement clotting factor is given or the procedure terminated
4. All of the above

Q30. Plasma volume and total blood volume calculations(TBV) are mentioned, which of them is true?

1. Blood volume is equal to 7% of the body weight and plasma corresponds to 1 minus the hematocrit (1 − hematocrit). So, the plasma volume is calculated = 0.07 (L/kg) × body weight (kg) × (1 − hematocrit)
2. The other method to calculate plasma volume: plasma volume (mL) = (1 − hematocrit) × (b + c × body weight [kg]) where b = 1,530 and c = 41.0 for males; and b = 864 and c = 47.2 for females
3. For total blood volume calculations; males, TBV (inL) = (0.3669*[height(in m)]^3) + 0.03219*[weight (in Kg)] + 0.6041; and females, TBV (ML = (0.3561*[height(in m)]^3 + (0.03308* [weight (in Kg)])+0.1833
4. All of the above

Q31. Which of the following is false in Nadler's formula?

1. Nadler's formula is a complex formula considering the height, bodyweight, and gender of a person
2. Most apheresis equipment uses this formula to calculate the TBV
3. This formula cannot be used for children <25 kg
4. None of the above

Q32. An accurate TBV is difficult to determine in children, yet it is preferred to use mL/kg according to the age group. Average TBVs in young children are mentioned and which of the following is false?

1. 89–105 mL/kg in premature infants
2. 82–86 mL/kg in term newborns
3. 73–82 mL/kg in infants and preschool children
4. None of the above

Q33. A patient who is recently diagnosed with thrombotic thrombocytopenic purpura is scheduled to undergo an urgent therapeutic plasma exchange procedure. This exchange will involve the replacement of 1.5 blood volumes. The patient's total blood volume is 5000ml, and their haematocrit level is 36%. What is the total volume of plasma that will be replaced in a single procedure?

1. 3135 ML
2. 3410 ML
3. 4800 ML
4. 5500 ML

Q34. Which of the following is false during processing of plasma volume?

1. One plasma volume is prescribed for removal of lipoprotein as it is primarily distributed intravascularly
2. One plasma volume is prescribed for removal of IgM because it is primarily distributed intravascularly
3. About 42% of IgA is intravascular
4. Both bilirubin and ammonia do not diffuse into the intracellular space

Q35. Which of the following is true for processing plasma volume?

1. The total processing volume for IgG removal is ideally 1.5 times the plasma volume
2. The Plasma exchange for removal of IgG is done every other day
3. IgG distributed in extravascular space is 55%
4. All of the above

Q36. Virus Removal and Eradication by Double Filtration Plasmapheresis (VRAD) is applied for chronic viral infection caused by

1. Hepatitis C type 1
2. Hepatitis C type 2
3. Hepatitis A
4. Hepatitis E

Q37. Virus Removal and Eradication by Double Filtration Plasmapheresis (VRAD) is practiced to achieve a viral free condition (sustainable viral response) when cases present with

1. HCV-RNA serotype 1 more than 100 kIU/mL infection and is resistant to Interferon alpha
2. HCV-RNA serotype 1more than 50 kIU/mL infection and is not resistant to Interferon alpha
3. HCV-RNA serotype 1more than 200 kIU/mL infection and is not resistant to Interferon alpha
4. HCV-RNA serotype 1more than 50 kIU/mL infection and is resistant to Interferon alpha

Q38. A maximum five procedures by DFPP is recommended for chronic HCV Infection within a period of

1. 5 days
2. 7 days
3. 8 days
4. 9 days

Q39. PEG-IFN is recommended on

1. On day 1 and 8 immediately after DFPP (usually within 1 h)
2. On Day 2 and 4 immediately after DFPP (usually within 1 h)
3. On day 8 and 9 immediately after DFPP (usually within 1 h)
4. Any of the above

Q40. DFPP is usually performed for HCV Infection prescribing a plasma processing dose of

1. 30ml/kg
2. 40ml/Kg
3. 50 ml/kg
4. 60 ml/kg

Q41. The following is true for VRAD (Virus Removal and Eradication by Double Filtration Plasmapheresis)?

1. The plasma separation is achieved by a plasma separator (1st filter, Plasma flo™ OP-08 W or equivalent)
2. 2nd filter (Cascade flo™ EC-50 W or equivalent) with a pore size of 30 nm prevents the re-entrance of viral particles with a diameter of 55–60 nm
3. The efficacy of the procedure is indicated by the reduction in HCV viral load of the patients which is based on the total processed plasma volume
4. All of the above

Q42. Which of the following is false for VRAD (Virus Removal and Eradication by Double Filtration Plasmapheresis)?

1. Virus Removal and Eradication by Double Filtration Plasmapheresis (VRAD) is limited by Serum Fibrinogen levels
2. Virus Removal and Eradication by Double Filtration Plasmapheresis (VRAD) is preferred as it is not limited by Serum Fibrinogen levels
3. The viral load of HCV from the liver is enormous; its generation rate is 10*12 virions per day and its half life is 2.7 h
4. Immediately after DFPP, there is a rebound phenomenon with respect to HCV

Q43. The following in Plasma Flo (OP-02W) is true?

1. Plasmaflo (OP-02W) is a *small-volume plasma separator* from Asahi Kasei Medical (Tokyo, Japan)
2. With Plasma Flo membrane, the Extra Corpuscular Volume (including plasma side) during a single Plasma Exchange is slightly less than 60 ml
3. It consists of Polyethylene (coated by ethylene-vinylalcohol copolymer) as the hollow fiber material
4. All of the above

Q44. Which of the following is true for Plasma Separator and Fractionator?

1. Plasma separator- Plasma flo
2. Plasma separator-Eva cure
3. Plasma fractionator-Eva flux
4. All of the above

Q45. All of the following are true in Prisma flex/Prismax except:

1. Prismaflex/Prismax are one of the few mTPE Kits that are USFDA approved
2. Both systems can be used in patients with body weight >20kgs
3. Both of them are used for CRRT
4. None of the above

Q46. All of the following are true except:

1. Cureflo-Continous Renal Replacement Therapy
2. Plasmaflo- low protein sieving coefficient and high protein loss
3. Cascadeflo-Maximum albumin loss
4. None of the above

Q47. All of the following is true in Rheopheresis except:

1. Rheopheresis is a semi-selective apheresis technique that varies from DFPP in terms of the secondary filter's properties
2. Fibrinogen, total and LDL cholesterol, triglycerides, lipoproteins, von Willebrand factor, alpha 2 macroglobulin, IgM, and other vascular risk factors (mw >60 kDa) can all be eliminated by the secondary filter
3. Because rheopheresis is known to improve hemorheology, it is not appropriate for the treatment of microcirculatory disorders marked by blood hyper viscosity
4. Rheopheresis is frequently advised for the treatment of diabetic foot, peripheral arterial disease, abrupt deafness, and age-related macular degeneration

Q48. Combination of Filtration and Centrifugation Techniques are used in plasmapheresis, which of the following is true?

1. By Autopheresis C™ (Fresenius Kabi) and Aurora™ (Fresenius Kabi)
2. Fresenius Kabi uses a spinning membrane, hence incorporates both membrane and centrifugation technology
3. This method is utilized for the collection of approximately 500-990 ml of plasma, it operates as an intermittent-flow system
4. All of the above

Q49. Which of the following is false with respect to FXIII in DFPP procedure?

1. There is a decrease of FXIII to 10–20% of normal values when DFPP is used
2. FXIII plays a role in cross bridging between fibrin molecules and also tightens the clot that results by means of coagulation cascade
3. A decrease to less than 1% of normal values of FXIII causes fatal bleeding
4. Fibrinogen and Factor XIII (FXIII) have a long half-life, ie a slow production rate, and hence repeated therapies will reduce the levels of these factors

ANSWERS

Q1. Ans(4)	**Q2.** Ans(4)	**Q3.** Ans(3)	**Q4.** Ans(4)	**Q5.** Ans(4)	**Q6.** Ans(4)
Q7. Ans(4)	**Q8.** Ans(1)	**Q9.** Ans(4)	**Q10.** Ans(4)	**Q11.** Ans(4)	**Q12.** Ans(4)
Q13. Ans(4)	**Q14.** Ans(4)	**Q15.** Ans(4)	**Q16.** Ans(4)	**Q17.** Ans(4)	

Q18. Ans(2) [*This membrane can selectively remove low and intermediate molecular weight albumin bound substances while retaining high molecular weight proteins such as fibrinogen and immunoglobulin M*]

Q19. Ans(4)	**Q20.** Ans(4)	**Q21.** Ans(4)	**Q22.** Ans(4)	**Q23.** Ans(4)	**Q24.** Ans(4)
Q25. Ans(4)	**Q26.** Ans(4)	**Q27.** Ans(4)	**Q28.** Ans(4)	**Q29.** Ans(4)	**Q30.** Ans(4)
Q31. Ans(4)	**Q32.** Ans(4)	**Q33.** Ans(3)	**Q34.** Ans(4)	**Q35.** Ans(4)	**Q36.** Ans(1)
Q37. Ans(1)	**Q38.** Ans(4)	**Q39.** Ans(1)	**Q40.** Ans(3)	**Q41.** Ans(4)	**Q42.** Ans(2)
Q43. Ans(4)	**Q44.** Ans(4)	**Q45.** Ans(4)	**Q46.** Ans(4)	**Q47.** Ans(3)	**Q48.** Ans(4)

Q49. Ans(3) [*A profound decrease of FXIII to less than 5% of normal values causes fatal bleeding*]

REFERENCES

1. Connelly-Smith L, Alquist CR, Aqui NA, Hofmann JC, Klingel R, Onwuemene OA, Patriquin CJ, Pham HP, Sanchez AP, Schneiderman J, Witt V, Zantek ND, Dunbar NM. Guidelines on the use of therapeutic apheresis in clinical practice—evidence-based approach from the writing Committee of the American Society for apheresis: the ninth special issue. J Clin Apher. 2023;38(2):77–278.
2. Noiri E. and Hanafusa N., The Concise Manual of Apheresis Therapy. Tokyo; Japan:Springer; 2014
3. Nadler SB, Hidalgo JH, Bloch T. Prediction of blood volume in normal human adults. Surgery. 1962;51:224–32.
4. Hulbert ML, Scothorn DJ, Panepinto JA, Scott JP, Buchanan GR, Sarnaik S, et al. Exchange blood transfusion compared with simple transfusion for first overt stroke is associated with a lower risk of subsequent stroke: a retrospective cohort study of 137 children with sickle cell anemia. J Pediatr. 2006;149(5):710–2.
5. Cohn, CS, Delaney M, Johnson ST, Katz LM, editors. Technical Manual, 20th ed Bethesda, MD: AABB, 2020.
6. Kaplan AA. A Practical Guide to Therapeutic Plasma Exchange. Malden, MA: Blackwell Science; 1999.
7. Reverberi, R., & Reverberi, L. Removal kinetics of therapeutic apheresis. *Blood Transfusion*, 2007;*5*(3), 164.
8. Yamashita T, Arai K, Sakai A, Mizukoshi E, Sakai Y, Kagaya T, Nakamoto Y, Honda M, Wada T, Yokoyama H, Kaneko S Virological effects and safety of combined double filtration plasmapheresis (DFPP) and interferon therapy in patients with chronic hepatitis C: a preliminary study. Hepatol Res 2006;36:167–175
9. Fujiwara K, Kaneko S, Kakumu S, Sata M, Hige S, Tomita E, Mochida S Virus Reduction Therapy Study Group. Double filtration plasmapheresis and interferon combination therapy for chronic hepatitis C patients with genotype 1 and high viral load. Hepatol Res 2007; 37:701–710
10. Soma I, Hattori M. Blood puri fi cation in children. In: Apheresis manual revised 3 version. Japanese Society for Apheresis, Syujunsya, 2010;pp 184–191 (in Japanese)
11. Winters JL, editor. Apheresis:principles and practice.4th ed. Vol.1, Therapeutic Apheresis. Bethesda, MD:AABB;2020
12. Nakanishi T, Suzuki N, Kuragano T, et al. Current topics in therapeutic plasmapheresis. Clin Exp Nephrol 2014;18:41–9. 10.1007/s10157-013-0838-0
13. Hepatitis C. Available: https://www.who.int/news-room/fact-sheets/detail/hepatitis-c
14. Ishikawa T, Abe S, Kojima Y, et al. Prediction of a sustained viral response in chronic hepatitis C patients who undergo induction therapy with double filtration plasmapheresis plus interferon-β/ribavirin. Exp Ther Med 2015;9:1646–50. 10.3892/etm.2015.2340

15. Kamimura H, Kamimura K, Tsuchiya A, Terai S. Successful treatment of positive-sense RNA virus coinfection with autoimmune hepatitis using double filtration plasmapheresis. BMJ Case Rep. 2021; 14(3):e236984.
16. *Ratti Ram Sharma, MD; Rekha Hans, MD and Divjot Singh Lamba, MD* TRANSFUSION MEDICINE TECHNICAL MANUAL Third Edition 2023.p184.
17. Kozanoglu I. *Problem Solving in Apheresis Medicine*, Switzerland:Springer Nature; 2024.
18. Blättler W, Straub PW, Jeanneret C, Horak GS. Effect of low fibrinogen concentrations on the rheology of human blood in vitro. Am J Physiol. 1979; 236((3)):H447–H450.]
19. Pulido J, Sanders D, Winters JL, Klingel RJ. Clinical outcomes and mechanism of action for rheopheresis treatment of age-related macular degeneration (AMD) J Clin Apher. 2005; 20((3)):185–194.
20. Pulido JS, Sanders D, Klingel R. Rheopheresis for age-related macular degeneration clinical results and putative mechanism of action. Can J Ophthalmol. 2005; 40((3)):332–340.]
21. Wild C, Mathis S, Guba B, Gartlehner G. Rheopheresis for age-related macular degeneration. Ophthalmologe. 2009; 106((2)):127–132.]
22. Valbonesi M, Mora F, Mora R, Carlier P. Rheopheresis for sudden hearing loss (SHL) Int J Artif Organs. 2004; 27((9)):806–809.
23. Balletshofer BM, Stock J, Rittig K, Lehn-Stefan A, Braun N, Burkart F, et al. Acute effect of rheopheresis on peripheral endothelial dysfunction in patients suffering from sudden hearing loss. Ther Apher Dial. 2005; 9((5)):385–390.
24. Weiss N. A critical review on the use of lipid apheresis and rheopheresis for treatment of peripheral arterial disease and the diabetic foot syndrome. Semin Dial. 2012;25((2)):220–227
25. Naciri Bennani H, Banza AT, Terrec F, Noble J, Jouve T, Motte L, Malvezzi P, Rostaing L. Cryoglobulinemia and double-filtration plasmapheresis: Personal experience and literature review. Ther Apher Dial. 2023; (1):159-169. Available from: http://dx.doi.org/10.1002/jca.21897
26. Jagdish K, Jacob S, Varughese S, David VG, Mohapatra A, Valson A, et al. Effect of double filtration plasmapheresis on various plasma components and patient safety: A prospective observational cohort study. Indian J Nephrol 2017;27:377-83
27. Siami GA, Siami FS. Current topics on cryofiltration technologies. Ther Apher. 2001; (4):283-6.

Chapter 5

THERAPEUTIC PLASMA EXCHANGE (TPE) IN NEUROLOGICAL DISORDERS

Dr. Swapna and Dr. Sunantha

Q1. Which of the following is an indication for First line therapy with plasma exchange?
1. Acute stroke secondary to Sickle Cell Disease
2. Stroke prophylaxis in non-acute Sickle Cell Disease
3. Chronic Inflammatory Demyelinating Polyneuropathy (CIDP)
4. All of the above

Q2. Which of the following is true in NMOSD (Neuromyelitis optica spectrum disorders)?
1. First-line therapy with plasma exchange is better than high-dose corticosteroid pulse therapy in achieving complete remission in *transverse myelitis* and not in optic neuritis
2. *Escalation therapy* with plasma exchange increases remission
3. Plasma exchange is effective in corticosteroid refractory *acute attacks* and often ineffective as a maintenance therapy
4. All of the above

Q3. Regarding Neuromyelitis Optica (NMO), the following is true
1. NMO is considered a variant of Multiple Sclerosis (an Asian optic spinal form of Multiple Sclerosis) in terms of clinical course and pathological characteristics
2. IgG1 autoantibodies to aquaporin4 (AQP4) water channel in sera of these patients indicates astrocyte impairment that can accompany the loss of AQP4
3. Apheresis is applied for removal of these antibodies
4. All of the above

Q4. Which of the following is true in Autoimmune encephalitis?
1. Plasma exchange (PE) when combined with corticosteroids and immunoglobulins fastens the remission
2. Plasma exchange (PE) is useful in autoimmune encephalitis as the titres of LGI1 and CASPR2 autoantibodies decrease and there is clinical improvement
3. The replacement fluid used in Plasma exchange (PE) is albumin
4. All of the above

Q5. Autoantibodies to voltage-gated potassium channels (VGKC) are removed by apheresis in
1. Isaac's syndrome
2. Reye's syndrome
3. Hemolytic Uremic Syndrome
4. Upshaw–Schulman syndrome

Q6. Autoantibodies to voltage-gated calcium channels (VGCC) are the target substances for removal by apheresis in
1. LEMS (Lambert–Eaton Myasthenic Syndrome)
2. Isaac's syndrome
3. Hemolytic Uremic Syndrome
4. Upshaw–Schulman syndrome

Q7. Which of the following is true in the treatment of Lambert–Eaton Myasthenic Syndrome (LEMS)?
1. LEMS is often complicated with *malignancies* (eg. small cell lung cancer)
2. *Nerve conduction studies* are useful for diagnosis
3. The *auto antibodies* hamper the acetyl choline release from presynaptic nerve terminals in *neuromuscular junctions* and they are removed by apheresis
4. All of the above

Q8. Which of the following is true for Apheresis in N-Methyl- D -Aspartate Receptor (NMDAR) Encephalitis?

1. NMDAR encephalitis is paraneoplastic encephalitis often accompanied by *ovarian teratoma*
2. *Symptoms* of NMDAR (psychiatric presentations, memory disturbance, involuntary movements, confusion, and convulsion) mostly improve with the removal of the ovarian teratoma
3. *Plasma Exchange* can be combined with *immunosuppressive therapy* and it is useful when started *early* in the course of NMDAR encephalitis
4. All of the above

Q9. In the history of Guillain Barre Syndrome, which of the following is true?

1. In 1859, Jean-Baptiste Octave Landry was the first to document a case of distal sensory "formications" accompanied by ascending weakness following a prodromal fever, malaise, and pain, which ultimately progressed to paralysis over a span of three weeks, resulting in death due to respiratory failure
2. Georges Guillain and Jean-Alexandre Barre subsequently reported two cases exhibiting albumin cytologic dissociation in cerebrospinal fluid (CSF) tests, and hence differentiated this syndrome from paralysis caused by poliomyelitis
3. Guillain-Barre-Strohl syndrome or Landry-Guillain-Barre-Strohl syndrome is more often, the Guillain-Barre syndrome (GBS) and is named in honour of the two *French* army neurologists
4. All of the above

Q10. Which among the following is false regarding TPE in Guillain Barre Syndrome GBS?

1. The technique of TPE was first introduced as a possible treatment for Guillain-Barre syndrome (GBS) in *1978*
2. Further *research* over the next few years found TPE significantly *beneficial* in treatment of Guillain Barre Syndrome (GBS)
3. By late 80s, TPE was extensively used as a *first line* treatment in the acute management of GBS
4. None of the above

Q11. Which of the following is true regarding therapeutic apheresis in GBS?

1. *IAPP* can be recommended for Guillain–Barre syndrome
2. The effect of therapeutic apheresis on *rapidly progressive or severe* Guillain–Barre syndrome is established
3. The modalities as (IVIG & Plasma Exchange) are of *little use* in patients with mild GBS, treatment failure, and treatment-related fluctuation
4. All of the above

Q12. Which of the following is true in management of GBS?

1. GBS, in 90% acute inflammatory demyelinating polyradiculoneuropathy, is immunologically mediated
2. The North American Guillain-Barre Study Group trial implied that the mechanical ventilation treatment was decreased by half with application of TPE (1985)
3. The Cochrane Neuromuscular Disease Group reported that TPE is effective and when ideally started within 7 days of disease onset
4. All of the above

Q13. Which of the following is false regarding the gangliosides of neuron?

1. Gangliosides, which are sphingolipids containing sialic acid, serve as significant components of neuronal membranes
2. The gangliosides are categorized as either simple or complex and are classified into various ganglio-series based on the quantity of sialic acids and the configuration of the oligosaccharide chain
3. GM1 is recognized as the most prevalent ganglioside found in the adult central nervous system (CNS)
4. GD3 is a complex ganglioside

Q14. Which of the following is true in the various types of GBS?

1. Acute inflammatory demyelinating polyneuropathy (*AIDP)(*first to be recognized over a century ago) is the most common form of GBS
2. In AIDP, the *immune* attack is directed at peripheral nerve myelin with secondary by-stander axon loss
3. *Axonal motor and sensorimotor variants* were described in the last 30 years and are mediated by *molecular mimicry* targeting peripheral nerve motor axons
4. All of the above

Q15. The target substances in Chronic Inflammatory Demyelinating Polyneuropathy include which of the following?

1. A*utoantibodies* against nodal and paranodal proteins
2. H*umoral* components of the immune system including TNF- α, IFN- γ
3. The others such as *inflammatory cytokines, adhesive molecules, and complement components*
4. All of the above

Q16. Which of the following is true in Chronic Inflammatory Demyelinating Polyneuropathy (CIDP)?

1. CIDP can occur in association with a *Monoclonal Gammopathy of Undetermined Signifi cance (MGUS)* and few other systemic illnesses
2. Autoantibodies to *myelin-associated glycoprotein* are detected in 50% of CIDP patients with IgM MGUS
3. Plasma Exchange is more efficacious for *IgA or IgG* gammopathy than IgM gammopathy
4. All of the above

Q17. Which of the following is true in Guillain–Barre Syndrome (GBS) regarding the target substance removal by apheresis?

1. Autoantibodies to ganglioside GM, GD1a, etc. (IgG, IgM, IgA) in case of *axonal* type of GBS are removed
2. Helps in removal of *immune complex and complement components*
3. Helps to cause s*uppression* of activated T cells
4. All of the above

Q18. Which among the following is true in the various types of Guillain–Barre Syndrome (GBS)?

1. In the *demyelinating type* GBS, injury begins from the myelin sheath of peripheral nerves
2. In *axonal type* GBS injury begins with axon and shows delayed recovery
3. *Campylobacter* infection often leads to axonal type GBS
4. All of the above

Q19. Which of the following is used as diagnostic criteria for GBS?

1. The *Brighton criteria* is used
2. It includes *clinical, cerebrospinal fluid* (CSF), and *electrophysiological* findings
3. CSF analysis shows *albumin cytological* dissociation
4. All of the above

Q20. Which of the following is true in GBS Variants?

1. Miller–Fischer syndrome (MFS) is a *variant form of GBS* with ataxia, areflexia and external ophthalmoplegia
2. *Anti-ganglioside GQ1b antibodies* (IgG) are present in the vast majority of patients with MFS variant of GBS
3. Apheresis is indicated for the treatment of a *MFS subpopulation* with GBS overlap
4. All of the above

Q21. Which of the following is false regarding the immunopathogenesis of GBS?

1. GBS results from *immune responses to non self* antigens (infectious agents, vaccines) that misdirect the host nerve tissue through a resemblance-of-epitope (molecular mimicry) mechanism
2. The *neural targets* are often the glycoconjugates (specifically gangliosides)
3. Antiganglioside antibodies (Anti-GQ1b), are seen in 20–50% of GBS (AMAN and AMSAN) cases, and preceded by *Campylobacter. jejuni* infection
4. *C. jejuni* strains also trigger activation of dendritic cells via signalling through Toll-like receptor 4 (TLR4), promoting B-cell differentiation and further amplifying humoral autoimmunity

Q22. Which of the following is false regarding the clinical presentation of GBS?

1. GBS manifests as a rapidly evolving *areflexic motor paralysis* with or without sensory disturbance
2. The common pattern is an ascending paralysis that is *first* noticed as *rubbery legs*
3. About *30%* of the affected patients require *ventilatory assistance* at some time during the illness
4. The most common preceding infection associated with Guillain-Barré syndrome is E.Coli

Q23. Which of the following is false regarding the treatment of GBS?

1. Either high-dose intravenous immune globulin (IVIg) or plasmapheresis (PLEX) are indicated, as they both are known to be equally effective for typical GBS
2. A combination of the two therapies is not significantly better than either of them when used alone
3. Plasma exchange is often the initial therapy chosen because of good safety record
4. IVIg is often the initial therapy chosen because of its ease of administration and good safety record

Q24. Label the therapeutic treatment modalities of GBS.

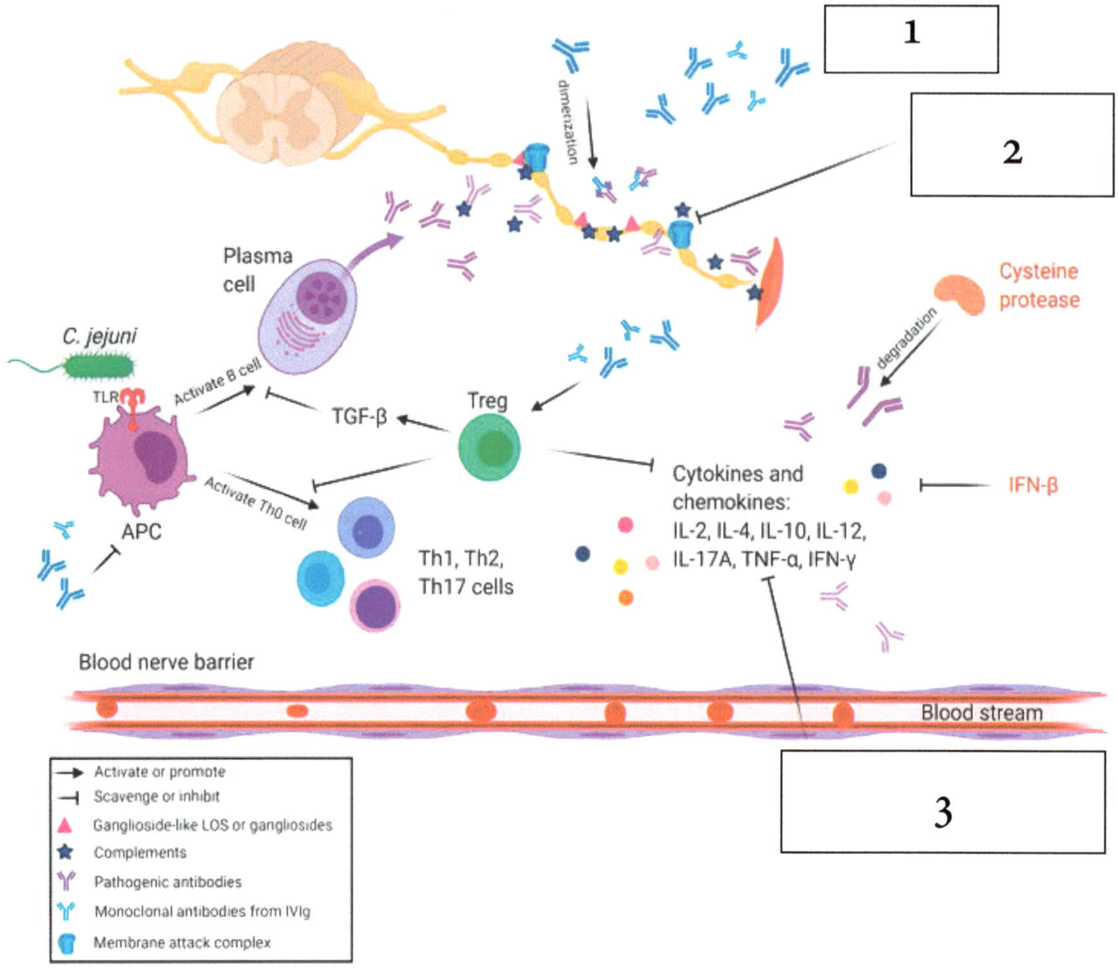

Fig V-1: Adapted from Shang et al. (18) 2021CCBY4.0

1. 1. Plasma Exchange, 2. IVIg, 3. Eculizumab
2. 1. IVIg, 2. Eculizumab, 3. Plasma Exchange
3. 1. IVIg, 2. Plasma Exchange, 3. Eculizumab
4. 1. Plasma Exchange, 2. Eculizumab, 3. IVIg

Q25. Which of the following is true regarding the ZIPPER method of TPE?

1. Zipper Method consists of implementation of plasmapheresis and IVIG in an *interpenetrating* manner
2. "Zipper method" was accompanied with subjectively *shorter ventilator times* and shorter hospitalisation
3. *It has been reported to have better outcomes* in few *pediatric* patients with severe GBS when compared to TPE or IVIG; or TPE plus IVIG approaches
4. All of the above

Q26. Which of the following is true regarding the anti-ganglioside antibodies testing in GBS?

1. AMAN (acute motor axonal neuropathy (AMAN))- anti-GM1 antibodies IgG polyclonal
2. AMAN (acute motor axonal neuropathy (AMAN))- Anti-GQ1b IgM antibodies
3. Miller Fischer syndrome- anti-GM1 antibodies IgM polyclonal
4. Miller Fischer syndrome- anti-GM1 antibodies IgA polyclonal

Q27. Which of the following is true with respect to Therapeutic Plasma Exchange (TPE) in GBS?

1. It is Category I Grade 1A (*ASFA category and rationale)*
2. TPE is beneficial in both the mildly and severely affected individuals; most of the patients are able to walk after 4 weeks
3. TPE is often helpful for additional relapses
4. All of the above

Q28. Which of the following is false regarding Plasma exchange therapy for GBS?
1. A course of PLEX usually consists of ~*40–50 mL/kg plasma exchange* 4–6 times over 7–12 days
2. TPE reduces the need for *mechanical ventilation* from 27 to 14%
3. TPE also increases the likelihood of *full recovery* at 1 year by from 55 to 68%
4. *Relapses* may occur in up to 25% to 30% of patients 2 to 3 weeks following treatment with TPE

Q29. Which of the following is true regarding IVIg therapy for GBS?
1. IVIg is usually administered as *five daily infusions* for a total dose of 2 g/kg body weight
2. GBS autoantibodies are neutralized by *anti-idiotypic antibodies* present in IVIg
3. TPE was reported to be more *cost-effective* in *India* than IVIG
4. All of the above

Q30. The immediate side effects of IVIG include:
1. Flu-like symptoms were reported in about 80% of the treated patients
2. Skin reactions were reported in about 6% of the treated patients
3. Cardiovascular and pulmonary reactions were seen in rare cases
4. All of the above

Q31. Which among the following are the delayed effects of IVIG?
1. *Renal and electrolyte effects* including *acute kidney injury* occur within10 days of IVIG; and peak at 5 days
2. *Hyponatremia, hypomagnesemia* occur any time during transfusion of IVIG; and recovery is *spontaneous*
3. *Neurological* reactions as *headache* (50%) starts 6–12 h after infusion and can last between 24-72 h
4. All of the above

Q32. Which of the following is false in management by IVIG infusion?
1. If patient is indicated for IVIG treatment, the *risk* is assessed and *laboratory tests* are done
2. *Premedications* such as anti-histaminics, steroids and anti-inflammatory drugs are included
3. When IVIG infusion is started, it is continued if tolerable or SCIg (Subcutaneous immunoglobulin) mode is tried or another brand is recommended
4. None of the above

Q33. Mechanism of action of IVIG in GBS are all of the following except
1. *Inhibiting* Fc-mediated activation of macrophages
2. Preventing the *binding of antibodies* to neural targets
3. Preventing *complement activation* which can trigger further nerve damage
4. *Scavenging* pathogens and autoimmune antibodies in patients' peripheral blood

Q34. Which of the following is true for the use of IVIG in neurology?
1. IVIG can be used in the *management* of intractable autoimmune epilepsy, paraneoplastic syndrome, autoimmune encephalitis, neuromyelitis optica
2. Subcutaneous immunoglobulin (SCIg) is newly emerging, and is a potential *future alternative*
3. The bioavailability of SCIg is lower when compared to IVIG but homeostatic level is more stable and both have *pharmacological equivalence*
4. All of the above

Q35. Mechanism of action of plasma exchange in GBS are all except
1. Removes *inflammatory cytokines* including TNF-α, IFN- γ, and IL-2
2. Removes *chemokines*
3. PE mainly functions *via* scavenging pathogens
4. Prevents the *binding of antibodies* to neural targets

Q36. Which of the following is true regarding Monoclonal Antibodies (mABs) as a treatment option for GBS?
1. mAbs are of IgG isotype which bind to the epitope of the target with their Fab antigen binding region, which results in specific function-inhibition or intracellular signalling
2. ANX005 (Tanruprubart) a humanized monoclonal antibody, is designed to inhibit C1q selectively, and hence prevents initiation of the classical complement cascade
3. Eculizumab is a humanized monoclonal IgG2 antibody against the complement protein C5
4. All of the above

Q37. All the drugs are currently in trial for treatment of GBS except

1. Eculizumab
2. Tanruprubart
3. Imflidase
4. Rituximab

Q38. Which of the following is false in GBS Variants?

1. Bickerstaff brainstem encephalitis (*BBE)* is a rare autoimmune neurological disorder first identified in 1951
2. The GBS Variants share clinical and immunological features with Guillain–Barré syndrome *(GBS)* and Miller–Fisher syndrome *(MFS)*
3. The *autoimmune encephalitis* is marked by sudden brainstem dysfunction, emerging a few days after an infection or vaccination
4. None of the above

Q39. Which of the following is true in Multiple Sclerosis (MS)?

1. The first study that focused on the effect of Therapeutic Plasma Exchange in MS patients was conducted *by Khatri et* al. in 1985
2. The first successful use of immunoadsorption (IA) in MS relapse was described in 2000 by *De Andrés et al.*
3. TPE is recommended by the American Society for Apheresis (ASFA) as *Grade II*
4. All of the above

Q40. One of the following methods/systems is used for treatment in multiple sclerosis

1. Hemophenix apparatus with ROSA nanomembrane
2. Immusorba TR-350
3. Prismaflex System
4. Glycosorba

Q41. The symptoms and mechanism of treatment for MS includes:

1. *Visual disturbances are* followed by different kind of symptoms such as paralysis of limbs, cerebellar ataxia, sensory disturbances, and bladder as well as rectal disturbances
2. The substances that are removed mainly are the *autoantibodies* to anti-myelin basic protein *(MBP*) and anti-myelin oligodendrocyte glycoprotein (*MOG*)
3. The substances as serum IgG, IgM *antibodies and complement* components are removed
4. All of the above

Q42. Which of the following is false regarding treatment therapy of MS?

1. IAPP is effective for *remitting-relapsing* multiple sclerosis (MS)
2. Apheresis is not efficacious for *chronic progressive* MS
3. A variety of treatments included are Interferon beta, immunosuppressants and steroids pulse therapy
4. None of the above

Q43. Which disease is classified as a Category I indication for Therapeutic Plasma Exchange (TPE)?

1) Myasthenia Gravis (MG)
2) Idiopathic inflammatory myopathies
3) Multiple Sclerosis
4) Lupus nephritis

Q44. Which one of the following is false with respect to TPE in MG?

1. The usefulness of TPE in MG was first described by *Pinching and Peter* in 1976
2. TPE directly removes *Ach Receptor antibodies*, and Anti-muscle specific tyrosine kinase *(MuSK)* antibody from circulation
3. There is emerging evidence that TPE also removes *low-density lipoprotein receptor-related* protein 4 positive *(LRP4+) in MG (present in 3% of the affected)*
4. None of the above

Q45. All of the following are true for MG and Myasthenic Crisis (MC) except:

1. MG has an annual incidence of *approximately 30 new cases per million*
2. About *15–20%* of the MG patients get into MC
3. According to the American Society for Apheresis, TPE is a well-established treatment for myasthenia exacerbation and myasthenic crisis *(Class III evidence, Category I)*
4. None of the above

Q46. All of the following are true with respect to different mechanisms of TPE for MG except:
1. Both *cTPE as well as mTPE* are used for MG
2. The *positive aspect of mTPE* is highlighted as the action completes in less than 24 h, preventing the development of any further antibodies during that time
3. Ideally mTPE is *rarely* recommended for MG
4. There are several classes of *antibiotics* that trigger MG exacerbations and hence it is important to re-evaluate antibiotic therapy

Q47. Which of the following is used for mTPE in MG?
1. Liposorba
2. Glycosorba
3. Prismaflex System (polypropylene hollow fibre prismafilter)
4. Prosorba

Q48. Which of the following is false regarding the Plasma Exchange for neurological disorders?
1. Immunoadsorption plasmapheresis *(IAPP)* is recommended for neurological disorders and has fewer side effects compared to plasma exchange *(PE)*
2. Double filtration plasmapheresis *(DFPP)* or plasma exchange *(PE)* are considered for non-responders to IAPP
3. PE is mainly practised in Europe and America
4. None of the above

Q49. For the treatment of MG, which of the following is true?
1. IAPP is recommended for anti-acetylcholine receptor antibody *(AchR)*-positive myasthenia gravis (MG)
2. DFPP is recommended for muscle-specific tyrosine kinase *(MuSK)*-positive MG
3. Patients who are *double-seronegative MG* (absence of both AChR and MuSK) may have autoantibodies to lipoprotein-related protein 4 (LRP4), ryanodine receptor, and titin
4. All of the above

Q50. Which of the following is true regarding sorbents and Anti-acetylcholine receptor (AchR) antibodies in MG?
1. Immusorba TR-350 ® containing tryptophan as a ligand is commonly used, and tryptophan has a high affinity for *anti-AchR antibodies* through hydrophobic interactions
2. Anti-acetylcholine receptor (AchR) antibodies are predominantly *IgG1 and IgG3 subclasses*
3. Anti-AchR antibodies are seen in *80% of patients with MG*, however the severity of the disease is *not* correlated with the plasma concentration of the antibodies
4. All of the above

Q51. Which of the following is true regarding treatment options in Myasthenia Gravis (MG)?
1. Both *TPE and IVIG* are applicable for MG Crisis
2. Apheresis is considered for *refractory cases* with systemic involvement, patients who do not tolerate glucocorticoids or immunosuppressants, and for *pre thymectomy* preparation
3. Clinical improvement is seen at the end of the third session of apheresis
4. All of the above

Q52. All of the following regarding the antibodies in MG is true except:
1. Anti-muscle specific tyrosine kinase (MuSK) antibodies are mainly *IgG4 subclass*
2. The *affinity* of the adsorption column of IAPP is *IgG subclass-dependent*
3. The affinity for *anti-MuSK antibodies* is much lower than that for anti-AchR antibodies often resulting in *desorption*
4. None of the above

Q53. MG is most often associated with
1. Thymic hyperplasia, thymoma and hyperthyroidism
2. Systemic lupus erythematosus
3. Rheumatoid arthritis
4. All of the above

Q54. TPE Category III and grade 2B is indicated for one of the following:
1. Sydenham's chorea, severe
2. PANDAS/PANS, exacerbation
3. Paraneoplastic Neurological Syndromes
4. Stiff Person Syndrome

Q55. Which of the following is true in acute disseminated encephalomyelitis (ADEM)?

1. TPE is Category II and Grade 2C
2. TPE removes pathogenic *autoantibodies as anti-MOG antibodies*
3. The differentiation of ADEM from a *first attack of multiple sclerosis* (MS) is important and has prognostic and therapeutic implications
4. All of the above

Q56. Which of the following is untrue regarding the replacement fluid 5% HAS:

1. It is manufactured from *cryo-depleted plasma*
2. *Transient reduction of clotting factors is a side effect* when administered
3. Nausea, flushing and rashes are potential adverse reactions, while *hypotension* is the most common
4. None of the above

Q57. Which of the following is false regarding the replacement fluids?

1. *Octaplas is a solvent-detergent (SD)*, virus-inactivated form of FFP which reduces risk of transfusion related infections and adverse reactions
2. Citrate toxicity (*hypocalcaemia*) symptoms are more common with FFP
3. TPE removes *60%* of clotting factors during an exchange and the risk of haemorrhage increases with longer duration of TPE
4. FFP is *NOT* given to replace clotting factors to reduce the bleeding risk especially when removal of vascath is required

ANSWERS

Q1. Ans(4)

Q2. Ans(4)

Q3. Ans(4)

Q4. Ans(4)

Q5. Ans(1)

Q6. Ans(1)

Q7. Ans(4)

Q8. Ans(4)

Q9. Ans(4)

Q10. Ans(4)

Q11. Ans(4)

Q12. Ans(4)

Q13. Ans(4)

Q14. Ans(4)

Q15. Ans(4)

Q16. Ans(4)

Q17. Ans(4)

Q18. Ans(4)

Q19. Ans(4)

Q20. Ans(4)

Q21. Ans(3)

The antibodies are Antiganglioside antibodies (*Anti-GM1)* seen in 20–50% of GBS (AMAN and AMSAN) cases, and preceded by *Campylobacter. jejuni* infection

Q22. Ans(4)

Cultural practices and seroepidemiologic methods indicate that 20-30% of all cases in North America, Europe, and Australia develop after an infection or reinfection with Campylobacter jejuni. A comparable percentage of cases is linked to infections from human herpes viruses, frequently CMV or Epstein-Barr virus. Additional viruses, such as HIV, hepatitis E, and Zika, as well as Mycoplasma pneumoniae, are also involved.

Q23. Ans(3)

Q24. Ans(2)

IVIg can reduce the production of harmful antibodies and pro-inflammatory substances released by activated T helper cells and B cells by acting on regulatory T cells (Tregs). IVIg also encourages the dimerization of antiganglioside antibodies and inhibits antigen-presenting cells (APCs) to mitigate immune responses. Plasma exchange (PE) primarily substitutes plasma rich in antiganglioside antibodies and pro-inflammatory substances with fresh frozen plasma or albumin. Nafamostat mesilate, Eculizumab and rEV576 are complement inhibitors that can stop the formation of the membrane attack complex (MAC).

Q25. Ans(4)

Q26. Ans(1)

The antibodies implicated are IgG (polyclonal) type; GM1 in Acute inflammatory demyelinating polyneuropathy (AIDP)

GD1a, GM1, GM1b, GalNac-GD1a in acute motor axonal neuropathy (AMAN)

GQ1b in Miller Fisher Syndrome (MFS)

GT1a in acute pharyngeal cervicobrachial neuropathy (APCBN)

Q27. Ans(4)

Q28. Ans(4)

Relapses may occur in up to 5-10% of patients 2 to 3 weeks following treatment with TPE

Q29. Ans(4)

Q30. Ans(4)

Q31. Ans(4)

Q32. Ans(4)

Q33. Ans(4)

Q34. Ans(4)

Q35. Ans(4)

Q36. Ans(4)

ANX005:

ANX005 (Tanruprubart), a human-derived monoclonal antibody, is engineered to selectively and completely inhibit C1q, thereby preventing the activation of the classical complement cascade. Inhibiting C1q at the beginning of the classical complement pathway reduces tissue inflammation and damage caused by downstream complement components, such as C3a and C5a (soluble anaphylatoxins that are highly inflammatory), C4b and C3b (signals for phagocytosis on cell surfaces), and C5b-9. Additionally, because C1q is the initial molecule in the complement system, the biological mechanisms of ANX005 are anticipated to remain consistent regardless of the patient's race, ethnicity, or geographic location.

Eculizumab:

Japanese Eculizumab Trial for GBS (JET-GBS)

This study was a 24-week, multi centre, double-blind, placebo-controlled, randomized phase 2 trial carried out in 13 hospitals throughout Japan. Individuals diagnosed with Guillain-Barré syndrome who were eligible for participation were aged 18 years or older and were unable to walk independently (Guillain-Barré syndrome functional grade 3–5). Participants were randomly allocated in a 2:1 ratio to receive 4 weeks of intravenous immunoglobulin along with either eculizumab (900 mg) or a placebo.

MAC formation is prevented by the complement inhibitors as Eculizumab, nafamostat mesilate, and rEV576. IFN-β attenuates inflammation induced by cytokines and chemokines. Cysteine protease degrades pathogenic antibodies and mitigates hyperreactive immune responses.

Q37. Ans(4)

Q38. Ans(4)

Q39. Ans(4)

Q40. Ans(1)

Q41. Ans(4)

Q42. Ans(4)

Q43. Ans(1)

Q44. Ans(4)

Q45. Ans(4)

Q46. Ans(3)

Q47. Ans(3)

Q48. Ans(4)

Q49. Ans(4)

Q50. Ans(4)

Q51. Ans(4)

Q52. Ans(4)

Q53. Ans(4)

Q54. Ans(1)

Q55. Ans(4)

Q56. Ans(4)

Q57. Ans(4)

FFP is given to replace clotting factors to reduce bleeding risk particularly when removal of vascath is required

REFERENCES

1. Arora N.; Procedures and Protocols in the Neurocritical Care Unit, Switzerland: Springer Nature;2022
2. Schwartz J, Padmanabhan A, Aqui N, Balogun RA, Connelly-SmithL, Delaney M, et al. Guidelines on the use of therapeuticApheresis in clinical practice-evidence-based approach from the writing Committee of the American Society for Apheresis: the seventh special issue. J Clin Apher. 2016;31(3):149–62.
3. Cortese I, Chaudhry V, So YT, Cantor F, Cornblath DR, Rae-GrantA. Evidence-based guideline update: plasmapheresis in neurologic disorders: report of the Therapeutics and Technology Assessment Subcommittee of the American Academy of Neurology. Neurology. 2011;76(3):294–300.
4. Kleiter I, Gahlen A, Borisow N, Fischer K, Wernecke KD, Wegner B, et al. Neuromyelitis optica: evaluation of 871 attacks and 1,153 treatment courses. Ann Neurol.2016;79(2):206–16.
5. Misu T, Fujihara K, Kakita A, Konno H, Nakamura M, WatanabeS, Takahashi T, Nakashima I, Takahashi H, Itoyama Y. Loss of aquaporin 4 in lesions of neuromyelitis optica: distinction from multiple sclerosis. Brain (a journal of neurology)130(Pt 5)2007;1224–1234.
6. Noiri E. and Hanafusa N., The Concise Manual of Apheresis Therapy. Tokyo: Springer Japan;2014
7. Osman C, Jennings R, El-Ghariani K, Pinto A. Plasma exchange in neurological disease. Pract Neurol. 2020;20(2):92–9.
8. Landry O. Note on acute ascending paralysis. Gaz Hebd Med Paris. 1859;6:4724.
9. Guillain G, Barré JA, Strohl A. On a syndrome of radiculoneuritis with hyperalbuminosis of the cerebrospinal fluid without cellular reaction. Remarks on the clinical and graphical characteristics of tendon reflexes. Bull Soc Med Hosp Paris. 1916;40:146270.
10. Vasques JF, de Jesus Gonçalves RG, da Silva-Junior AJ, Martins RS, Gubert F, Mendez-Otero R. Gangliosides in nervous system development, regeneration, and pathologies. Neural Regen Res. 2023;18(1):81.
11. Dimachkie MM, Barohn RJ. Guillain-Barré syndrome and variants. Neurol Clin. 2013 May;31(2):491-510.
12. Pascual-Goñi E, Martín-Aguilar L, Querol L. Autoantibodies in chronic inflammatory demyelinating polyradiculoneuropathy. Curr Opin Neurol. 2019 Oct;32(5):651-657.
13. Kesici S, Tanyıldız M, Yetimakman F, Bayrakci B. A Novel Treatment Strategy for Severe Guillain-Barré Syndrome: Zipper Method. J Child Neurol. 2019 Apr;34(5):277-283.
14. Hauser SL, Amato AA. Guillain-Barré syndrome (GBS). In: Jameson JL, Fauci AS, Kasper DL, Hauser SL, Longo DL, Loscalzo J, editors. *Harrison's principles of internal medicine*. 22nd ed. New York: McGraw-Hill Education; 2025.
15. Connelly-Smith L, Alquist CR, Aqui NA, Hofmann JC, Klingel R, Onwuemene OA, Patriquin CJ, Pham HP, Sanchez AP, Schneiderman J, Witt V, Zantek ND, Dunbar NM. Guidelines on the Use of Therapeutic Apheresis in Clinical Practice - Evidence-Based Approach from the Writing Committee of the American Society for Apheresis: The Ninth Special Issue. J Clin Apher. 2023 Apr;38(2):77-278. doi: 10.1002/jca.22043. PMID: 37017433. J Clin Apher. 2023;38:77–278.
16. Guo Y, Tian X, Wang X, Xiao Z. Adverse effects of immunoglobulin therapy. Front Immunol. 2018;
17. Chen Y, Wang C, Xu F, Ming F, Zhang H. Efficacy and tolerability of intravenous immunoglobulin and subcutaneous immunoglobulin in neurologic diseases. Clin Ther. 2019;41(10):2112–36.
18. Shang P, Feng J, Wu W, Zhang HL. Intensive Care and Treatment of Severe Guillain–Barré Syndrome. Frontiers in Pharmacology [Internet]. 2021 Apr 27;12(608130) p.6. Available from: https://www.ncbi.nlm.nih.gov/pmc/articles/PMC8113987/pdf/fphar-12-608130.pdf
19. Misawa S, Kuwabara S, Sato Y, Yamaguchi N, Nagashima K, Katayama K, et al. Safety and efficacy of eculizumab in Guillain-Barré syndrome: a multicentre, double-blind, randomised phase 2 trial. The Lancet Neurology [Internet]. 2018 Jun 1;17(6):519–29. Available from: https://pubmed.ncbi.nlm.nih.gov/29685815
20. Gorson KC. Evolving understanding of Guillain–Barré syndrome pathophysiology and the central role of the classical complement pathway in axonal injury. *Front Neurol.* 2025;16: 1572949.
21. Wiegers EJA, Jacobs BC. New insights in the immune treatment of Guillain-Barré syndrome. Current opinion in neurology [Internet]. 2025 Summer;10.1097/WCO.0000000000001408. Available from: https://pubmed.ncbi.nlm.nih.gov/40748027/
22. https://www.neurologylive.com/view/positive-phase-2-analyses-highlight-therapeutic-potential-imlifidase-guillain-barr-syndrome
23. Abide Z, Sif Nasr K, Kaddouri S, et al. Bickerstaff brainstem encephalitis: a case report. Radiol Case Rep 2023;18: 2704–06.
24. Faheem MSB, Zeeshan N, Atta Ur Rafe S, Samadi S. Bickerstaff encephalitis: a comprehensive narrative review of pathophysiology, clinical features, and global health considerations. Ann Med Surg (Lond). 2025; 87(8):5122-5131.
25. Bunganic, R., Blahutova, S., Revendova, K. *et al.* Therapeutic plasma exchange in multiple sclerosis patients with an aggressive relapse: an observational analysis in a high-volume center. *Sci Rep* 2022;**12**, 18374

26. de Andrés, C. & Giménez-Roldán, S. *Plasma immunoadsortion treatment of malignant multiple sclerosis with severe and prolonged relapses Genetics of Narcolepsy with Cataplexy View project History of Neurology View project.*
27. Tonev, D., & Momchilova, A. (2023). Therapeutic Plasma Exchange and Multiple Sclerosis Dysregulations: Focus on the Removal of Pathogenic Circulatory Factors and Altering Nerve Growth Factor and Sphingosine-1-Phosphate Plasma Levels. *Current Issues in Molecular Biology*, *45*(10), 7749-7774.
28. Skeie GO, Apostolski S, Evoli A, Gilhus NE, Illa I, Harms L, et al. Guidelines for treatment of autoimmune neuromuscular transmission disorders. Eur J Neurol. (2010) 17:893–902. 10.1111/j.1468-1331.2010.03019.x
29. Barth D, Nabavi Nouri M, Ng E, Nwe P, Bril V. Comparison of IVIg and PLEX in patients with myasthenia gravis. Neurology. (2011) 76:2017–23.10.1212/WNL.0b013e31821e5505
30. Pinching AJ, Peters DK. Remission of myasthenia gravis following plasma-exchange. Lancet. 1976;2:1373–6.
31. Dogra, A., Rana, K., Rathod, C., & Prakash, S. Outcome of therapeutic plasma exchange in Myasthenia gravis patients. *Journal of Family Medicine and Primary Care*,2020; *9*(12), 5971.
32. Kurnia D, Manggala SK, Irawany V. The role of therapeutic plasma exchange using membrane plasma separation in the late onset myasthenia gravis crisis: a case report. Anaesth. pain intensive care 2024;28(5):969–973.
33. Kohli R, Geneen LJ, Brunskill SJ, Doree C, Estcourt L, Chee SEJ, et al. Assessing efficacy and safety of replacement fluids in therapeutic plasma exchange: A systematic scoping review of outcome measures used. J Clin Apheresis. 2022;37(5):438–48.
34. Basic-Jukic N, Kes P, Glavas-Boras S, Brunetta B, Bubic-Filipi L, Puretic Z. Complications of therapeutic plasma exchange: Experience with 4857 treatments. Ther Apher Dial. 2005;9(5):391–5.
35. Howell C, Douglas K, Cho G, El-Ghariani K, Taylor P, Potok D, et al. Guideline on the clinical use of apheresis procedures for the treatment of patients and collection of cellular therapy products. Transfus Med. 2015;25(2):57–78.
36. CADTH CA for D and T in H. Octaplas compared with fresh frozen plasma to reduce the risk of transmitting lipid-enveloped viruses: an economic analysis and budget impact analysis. Vol. 1. Canadian Agency for Drugs and Technologies in Health; 2010.
37. Okafor C, Ward DM, Mokrzycki MH, Weinstein R, Clark P, Balogun RA. Introduction and overview of therapeutic apheresis. J Clin Apheresis. 2010;25(5):240–9.
38. Verboon C., Doets A. Y., Galassi G., Davidson A., Waheed W., Pereon Y., et al. (2019). Current treatment practice of Guillain–Barre syndrome. Neurology 93, e59–e76. 10.1212/wnl.0000000000007719
39. Guillain-Barre Syndrome Study Group. Plasmapheresis and guillain-barre syndrome. Neurology. 1985; 35: 1096–104.
40. Chevret S, Hughes RAC, Annane D. Plasma exchange for Guillain-Barre syndrome. Cochrane Database Syst Rev. 2017; 2(2):CD001798.

Chapter 6

THERAPEUTIC PLASMA EXCHANGE (TPE) IN HAEMOTOLOGICAL DISORDERS

Dr. Swapna, Dr. Priyanka and Dr. HariPriya

Q1. Which of the following is true in the history of Thrombotic thrombocytopenic purpura (TTP)?

1. Rubinstein was the first one to successfully treat a child with aTTP with exchange transfusion in 1959
2. Bukowski hypothesized that the success of plasma exchange was related to the removal of a soluble toxic substance in the plasma of aTTP patients
3. Bukowski had also successfully treated two aTTP patients with PE alone and hence supported the hypothesis
4. All of the above

Q2. According to ASFA guidelines, which condition is classified as Category I for Therapeutic Plasma Exchange (TPE) and it also serves as the major therapeutic intervention?

1. Warm autoimmune hemolytic anemia
2. Cryoglobulinemia
3. Thrombotic Thrombocytopenic Purpura (TTP)
4. Acquired Aplastic Anemia

Q3. All of the following are true regarding TTP except:

1. The mechanism of deficiency in immune TTP is caused by acquired autoantibodies against ADAMTS-13
2. In the congenital TTP, severe deficiency of ADAMTS-13 is recessively inherited
3. About less than 5% of all cases of TTP are congenital TTP (cTTP)
4. None of the above

Q4. Therapeutic Plasma Exchange is initiated in TTP only in patients with ADAMTS13 activity

1. <5%
2. <10%
3. <15%
4. <20%

Q5. Total plasma exchange is performed for TTP preferably within

1. 24 hours
2. 12 hours
3. 4-8hours
4. Anytime

Q6. The justification to begin total plasma exchange in a patient with TTP include

1. Microangiopathic hemolytic anemia (schistocytes, elevated lactate dehydrogenase (LDH) level, and indirect hyperbilirubinemia)
2. Thrombocytopenia
3. The absence of other conditions such as disseminated intravascular coagulation, malignant hypertension
4. All of the above

Q7. Plasma Exchange with fresh frozen plasma (FFP) as a replacement solution improved the mortality rate to <20% from the high mortality rate of

1. >90%
2. >80%
3. >70%
4. >60%

Q8. According to the recent International Society of Thrombosis and Hemostasis (ISTH) TTP guidelines,
1. FFP is typically administered at 10 to 15 mL/kg at three weekly intervals as maintenance therapy
2. FFP is administered daily for symptomatic patients until *symptoms resolve*
3. FFP is administered daily for symptomatic patients until *platelet counts* normalize
4. All of the above

Q9. All of the following are true regarding TTP except:
1. In 1998, deficiency of ADAMTS13 (a disintegrin and metalloprotease with thrombospondin type 1 repeats, member13), a von Willebrand factor-cleaving protease, was recognized as the cause of TTP
2. Thrombotic thrombocytopenic purpura is a medical emergency, and proper recognition is important because of the high mortality rates
3. Upshaw–Schulman syndrome is cTTP
4. In cTTP, severe deficiency of ADAMTS-13 does not manifest in neonates

Q10. Recombinant ADAMTS13 use is approved as treatment for the following type of TTP
1. Congenital
2. Acquired
3. Both of the above
4. None of the above

Q11. Congenital TTP is a microangiopathic disorder treated with
1. FFP, Factor VIII
2. Recombinant ADAMSTS 13
3. Caplacizumab
4. All of the above

Q12. Which of the following is false regarding IVIG use in TTP?
1. History begins in 1981, when Imbach et al. reported that when high-dose IVIG was used in 4 children with refractory immune thrombocytopenic purpura, patient's symptoms significantly improved and platelet count increased
2. The patients platelet counts were maintained at normal levels with IVIG infusion every 1 to 3 weeks and subsequently a series of cases treated with IVIG had shown good success
3. These unique findings facilitated the development of new treatment strategies for other autoimmune diseases
4. None of the above

Q13. The patients presenting with the *classic Moschcowitz's pentad* of microangiopathic hemolytic anemia, thrombocytopenia, neurologic abnormalities, fever, and kidney disease in TTP are
1. 10-20%
2. 20-30%
3. 30-40%
4. 40-50%

Q14. The *Triad* of haemolytic anaemia, thrombocytopenia, and acute kidney injury in Hemolytic Uraemic Syndrome is called
1. Gradenigos triad
2. Gasser's triad
3. Mackler's triad
4. Charcoat ′s triad

Q15. Which of the following is true for ADAMTS-13 activity in TTP?
1. Significantly decreased ADAMTS-13 activity, absence of ADAMTS-13 inhibitor is characteristic of Upshaw–Schulman syndrome
2. Decreased ADAMTS-13 activity, most cases with ADAMTS-13 inhibitor is seen in Drug-induced TTP (ticlopidine/ clopidogrel) and iTTP
3. Almost normal ADAMTS-13 activity (some cases with mildly decreased ADAMTS-13 activity) is seen in TTP associated with Hematopoietic stem cell transplantation
4. All of the above

Q16. Which of the following is true in the treatment of TTP?

1. Dr. Moschcowitz gave the first description of the disease TTP in 1924
2. Caplacizumab, steroids, plasma exchange, rituximab, and intravenous immunoglobulins (CASPERI) were used in aTTP
3. *Relapsed TTP* is defined as a recurrence of disease after 30 days from discontinuation of TPE
4. All of the above

Q17. Which of the following is true in management of TTP?

1. Acquired autoimmune TTP refers to the presence of autoantibodies against ADAMTS13 with an annual incidence of 3–11 cases per million people
2. Treatment with caplacizumab (an anti-vWF domain A1 nanobody), indicated faster normalization of the platelet count
3. TPE with *FFP* is *not* performed in TTP patients when patients are allergic to plasma or will avoid it due to religious reasons
4. All of the above

Q18. TPE is required daily in which of the following cases?

1. Hyperviscosity
2. TTP
3. Goodpasture syndrome
4. All of the above

Q19. Which of the following is false regarding the scores?

1. In 2010, Bentley et al. published the first clinical diagnostic tool for TTP
2. The French score was described by Coppo et al. in 2010, an alternative scoring system for identifying TTP
3. The plasmic score was developed by Bendapudi et al in 2014
4. None of the above

Q20. In TTP, the following is true except:

1. The PLASMIC score helps in distinguishing TTP from other Thrombotic Microangiopathys (TMAs)
2. Fewer number of plasma exchanges and shorter hospital stays was observed when caplacizumab was included in the treatment protocol
3. *Refractory TTP* is defined as a failure of platelet response after 4–7 days of plasmapheresis or a clinical deterioration despite the standard therapy
4. None of the above

Q21. The superiority of the clinical scores in assessing aTTP

1. Bentley Score>French Score>Plasmic Score
2. Bentley Score<French Score<Plasmic Score
3. Plasmic Score >Bentley Score>French Score
4. Plasmic Score <Bentley Score<French Score

Q22. The PLASMIC Score includes seven parameters; all of the following are included except:

1. Platelet counts
2. Creatinine
3. Markers of Haemolysis
4. Serum calcium

Q23. The risk stratification in PLASMIC Score includes:

1. Low risk: 0-4
2. Intermediate risk: 5
3. High risk:6-7
4. All of the above

Q24. The French score includes all except:

1. Platelet count
2. Serum Creatinine
3. Antinuclear antibody
4. Bilirubin

Q25. The diagnosis of TTP includes all of the following except:

1. ADAMTS13 activity test plays a role in the diagnosis
2. The ADAMTS13 tests including ADAMTS13 activity, inhibitors, or anti-ADAMTS13 IgG play a role in starting a patient on treatment with TPE and corticosteroids
3. Alternative diagnoses should always be sought in patients with plasma ADAMTS13 activity between 10 and 20 IU/dL (or 10-20% of normal)
4. None of the above

Q26. VITT-Vaccine induced Immune Thrombocytopenia is treated by

1. Anticoagulation
2. Upfront high- dose IVIg
3. Patients refractory to high- dose IVIg will require plasma exchange
4. All of the above

Q27. Plasma, cryoprecipitate reduced, is indicated in

1. Volume expansion
2. TTP
3. Drug Intoxication
4. Disseminated Intravascular Coagulation

Q28. The following drugs are known to cause TTP:

1. Cyclosporine
2. Tacrolimus
3. Mitomycin C
4. All of the above

Q29. Which of the following is true in diagnosis and treatment of TTP?

1. The Differential diagnosis TTP/TMA includes Malignant hypertension, DIC (secondary to sepsis, toxaemia of pregnancy, etc.)
2. The Differential diagnosis TTP/TMA also includes Vasculitis, Autoimmune disease (SLE, Rheumatoid arthritis), Catastrophic antiphospholipid syndrome
3. Several sessions of Plasma exchange are performed after the markers of normalization and recovery are seen
4. All of the above

Q30. A 32-year-old female patient, 6 weeks postpartum, and with no relevant medical history presents to the emergency department complaining about the presence of fatigue, petechiae, and dark- coloured urine during the last 2 days. Laboratory tests at admission indicate a white blood cell count of 11,100/mL, haemoglobin level of 7.1g/dL, and a platelet count of 38,000/mL. Serum electrolytes are normal except for increased creatinine at 2.6mg/dL. Urinalysis is positive haemoglobinuria, without erythrocytes. Lactate dehydrogenase (LDH) has increased to four times normal limit. A blood film indicates anaemia, schistocytes, helmet cells, fragmented red cells, thrombocytopenia. The ED physician intends to initiate urgent plasma exchange due to a suspected diagnosis of thrombotic thrombocytopenic purpura (TTP). Which laboratory test confirms the diagnosis of TTP?

1. ADAMTS13 level drawn prior to plasma exchange
2. ADAMTS13 level drawn immediately after plasma exchange
3. ADAMTS13 level drawn 24 h after the first procedure but immediately prior to the second procedure
4. Complement levels drawn prior to plasma exchange and after plasma exchange

Q31. After five sessions of plasma exchanges in a case of TTP, the patient's platelet count began to increase and it is 125,010/µL while LDH is now normal. However, the serum creatinine continues to increase to 4.3 mg/dL. What is the optimal step of management?

1. Carry on plasma exchange with no further modifications
2. Carry on with the plasma exchange with 1.5 plasma volumes rather than 1 plasma volume
3. Use cry depleted plasma instead of standard plasma in doing plasma exchange
4. Cessation of plasma exchange and the start of rituximab and vincristine

Q32. A 53-year-old previously healthy man with no significant past medical history is referred to his primary care physician with complaints of dull headaches and subjective fevers over the past few days. Routine laboratory investigations are obtained with the following results:

Complete Blood Count: Hgb: 12.7gms/dl, WBC: 6.8k cells/cu.mm Hct: 36.0%

Coagulation Profile:

PT: 13.6 secs
INR: 0.98
PTT: 36.2 secs

Chemistries

Na: 133 mmol/L
K: 3.7 mmol/L
Cl: 98 mmol/L
CO2: 29
BUN: 23 mg/dl
Cr: 0.90 mg/dl
Glu: 123 gms/dl

Peripheral Blood Smear showed thrombocytopenia, anisocytosis and hemolysis with schistocytes and micro spherocytes; reticulocytosis anemia

1. Begin emergent plasmapheresis with FFP replacement
2. Begin emergent plasmapheresis with albumin replacement
3. Transfuse 2 units of FFP, send an ADAMTS-13 activity to a reference lab, and wait for the results before considering plasmapheresis
4. Transfuse one unit of platelets and perform a 10-60 minute post-transfusion CBC

Q33. A 29-year-old female patient has been referred for TTP. She exhibits altered mental status, and her laboratory results show a haematocrit of 24.0, a platelet count of $23 \times 10^9/l$, and an LDH level of 3450 units/ml. Her weight is 72 kgs. What TPE regimen would you suggest? An aggressive TPE regimen is essential in this situation, as it poses a life-threatening risk. A standard regimen would consist of exchanging 1.5 plasma volumes daily for a period of 10–14 days. After this duration, further TPE is recommended based on the platelet count, plasma LDH levels, and the patient's clinical condition. Which of the following statements regarding the prescription is inaccurate?

1 plasma volume is $0.07\times 72 \times 0.76 = 3.83$ L;1.5 plasma volumes is 5.75 L

So the prescription would be:

1. Remove 5.75 L
2. Replace with 3.25L of 5% Albumin 2.0L of NS 0.5L of FFP
3. Premedicate with oral calcium
4. Give 10 ml of 10% calcium gluconate IV over the TPE session

Q34. A 32- year old man with a chronic myelogenous leukemia history in blast crisis with a white blood cell count of 400,500/ uL of which 97 percent are blasts. He is complaining of visual disturbances and pain in the chest. It is a planned intervention of therapeutic leukapheresis, and the apheresis team resolves to undertake the process under red blood cell-primed circuit. Which are the clues to conducting a red blood cell (RBC) prime in an apheresis procedure? (Select all that apply.)

1. Anemia
2. Ethylene tetroxide
3. High extracorporeal volume
4. Hydroxyethlstarch

Q35. The patient is a 23-year-old female with known history of sickle cell disease (SCD) whose left-sided paralysis has started about 1 hour before the arrival in the emergency department. Her husband informs that she is 12 weeks pregnant. She did not experience any SCD complications during the last two years but has a history of blood transfusion in her childhood. The acute ischemic stroke is evidenced by a non-contrast CT scan of the head. The physician in the emergency department consults on the application of red blood cell exchange (RBCx) in its management. What is the advice concerning the application of RBC exchange in this patient?

1. RBCx is not indicated to treat acute stroke in sickle cell disease
2. RBCx is contraindicated due to her pregnancy
3. RBCx should be performed as soon as possible due to the acute stroke
4. RBCx cannot be performed until after the hemoglobin S level is determined by hemoglobin electrophoresis

Q36. A 46-year-old female patient comes to the hospital with the complaints of a severe headache (8/10) and dyspnea with a respiratory rate of 26 breaths per minute and oxygen saturation of 87% on the room air. Her prescribed drugs are aspirin 81 mg a day and a multivitamin. Diffuse interstitial infiltrates without pneumonia are seen in the Chest X-ray. The CT head demonstrates the absence of acute ischemic or hemorrhagic abnormalities. Within a short period after imaging, the patient is agitated and confused. The laboratory assessment shows 186 × 10^9 /L of white blood cells. What is the immediate cause of clinical presentation of this patient?

1. Thrombotic stroke
2. Infection with Neisseria meningitidis
3. Leukostasis
4. Dementia

Q37. In the context of hyperleukocytosis and its role in Acute Promyelocytic Leukemia (APL), what caution is advised regarding the application of Leukocytapheresis in patients diagnosed with Acute Promyelocytic Leukemia (APL)?

1. Leukocytapheresis is the preferred first-line treatment for APL due to high thrombosis risk
2. Leukocytapheresis in APL may contribute to premature mortality
3. Leukocytapheresis should only be performed in APL if the WBC count exceeds 400 × 10^9/L
4. Central catheter placement must always be performed prior to Leukocytapheresis in APL patients

Q38. In patients with acute myeloid leukaemia (AML) complicated by leukostasis, when is it recommended to discontinue leukocytapheresis?

1. When the White Blood Cell (WBC) count drops below 400 × 10^9/L
2. When the WBC count drops below 100 × 10^9/L
3. When symptoms resolve and/or WBC count drops below 50 × 10^9/L
4. After a fixed course of 5 procedures.

Q39. A patient who has hemoglobin SC disease will present with acute ischemic stroke, and an automated red blood cell exchange will be requested. HbS and HbC are at 52 and 40 percent in the baseline hemoglobin fractions of the patient. You call the blood bank and order HbS negative, Rh- and Kell-compatible red blood cells. What are the target percentages of hemoglobin (Hb) percentages to be used when determining the fraction of cells remaining (FCR) of the exchange procedure? Post the American Society of Apheresis (ASFA) guidelines, what are the desired hemoglobin percentages?

1. HbS%<30%
2. HbC%<30%
3. HbS%<30% & HbC%<30%
4. HbS%<50%

Q40. A hemoglobin S/B 0 -thalassemia patient is receiving chronic automated red blood cell exchange secondary stroke prophylaxis. Before an exchange session is scheduled, a complete blood count (CBC) and hemoglobin electrophoresis are done in order to identify the exchange targets. Microcytosis is evidenced in the CBC. HbS 35% and HbA 2 4.3% (elevated) and a new peak in C zone are observed by hemoglobin electrophoresis at 3%. Which is the most probable explanation to these results?

1. The patient has beta globin tetramers due to thalassemia
2. The patient has underlying hemoglobin C trait
3. The patient received a unit from someone with hemoglobin C trait
4. The patient has alpha globin tetramers due to thalassemia

Q41. A 6-year-old male patient with transfusion-dependent B -thalassemia is hospitalized in a local children hospital, and the patient comes to the emergency department with fever and chills. His traveling abroad is non existent. Further history According to his care givers indicates he has a cyclic pattern of fever that has developed within 9 days of his last red blood cell transfusion. The Plasmodium species ring forms are evidenced by peripheral blood smear, which is also in line with transfusion-transmitted malaria. Red blood cell exchange is one of the management recommendations made by the fellow infectious disease. Based on American Society of Apheresis (ASFA) guiding principles, what is the current category and grade of recommendation of red blood cell exchange in malaria?
1. Category I grade I A
2. Category II grade II B
3. Category III grade I B
4. Category III grade IIB

Q42. Hereditary hemochromatosis (HH) is a genetic disease that is associated with iron overload caused by excessive absorption of iron and deposits iron in various organs. HH is developed due to several well described genetic mutations. HH is treated by way of therapeutic phlebotomy or in few situations automated red blood cell exchange. Which of these statements is correct when it comes to the question of the use of red blood cell exchange in the treatment of hereditary hemochromatosis?
1. Hereditary hemochromatosis is an ASFA category IV indication for red blood cell exchange
2. Red blood cell exchange can lower overall iron stores but has not been shown to reduce ferritin levels
3. Red blood cell exchange is significantly cheaper when comparing consumables to therapeutic phlebotomy
4. Red blood cell exchange results in fewer number of procedures and longer intervals between treatments when compared to therapeutic phlebotomy

Q43. What is the recommended therapeutic apheresis procedure in the treatment of hyperleukocytosis with clinical leukostasis, and what category of ASFA?
1. Red Cell Exchange (RCE), Category I
2. Leukapheresis, Category I
3. Therapeutic Plasma Exchange (TPE), Category III
4. Extracorporeal Photopheresis (ECP), Category II

Q44. The treatment of Multiple Myeloma includes:
1. Apheresis/PE for removing serum free light chains and M proteins
2. Plasma exchanges when cast nephropathy is proved by renal biopsy
3. The hematopoietic stem-cell transplantation along with chemotherapy will help in slow production of light chains
4. All of the above

Q45. Abnormal levels of the following are responsible for hyper viscosity in multiple myeloma
1. IgA
2. IgG3
3. k-light chains
4. All of the above

Q46. Which of the following is true for Multiple Myeloma regarding proteins?
1. The monomers of IgG, IgD, IgE, and the dimer of IgA are smaller compared to IgM a pentamer
2. When the total number of immunoglobulin molecules increases, it causes hyper viscosity syndrome
3. Hyper viscosity syndrome is triggered by an increase in serum proteins that can raise the viscosity of the plasma
4. All of the above

Q47. Double filtration plasmapheresis is useful in Multiple Myeloma when
1. The patients do not have impaired liver synthetic capacity
2. There is no abnormal haemostatic system
3. Fresh frozen plasma (FFP) is not needed or accepted by the patients
4. All of the above

Q48. The following is true for treatment of Multiple Myeloma:
1. The molecular weight of IgM is large, hence a large pore size membrane (such as EC-40W) is used as a secondary filter to remove IgM (DFPP)
2. The goal of plasma exchange (PE) is to prevent acute renal failure and to reduce light chains in myeloma patients
3. In patients with hyper viscosity syndrome, the goal of treatment/PE is to improve the symptoms
4. All of the above

Q49. A 69-year-old man with a known history of Waldenström macroglobulinemia presents to the emergency department with recent-onset blurry vision and headaches. Neurologic examination is notable for horizontal nystagmus. Laboratory evaluation reveals a serum viscosity of 6 centipoise (normal ≈ 1.5 cP) and an IgM level of 5.8 g/dL, both markedly elevated. The patient ́s symptoms are consistent with hyper viscosity syndrome. What is the most appropriate immediate management for this patient?

1. Perform emergent therapeutic plasma exchange (TPE) to rapidly remove IgM and relieve hyper viscosity-related symptoms
2. Initiate chemotherapy for Waldenström macroglobulinemia; if hyper viscosity-related symptoms do not improve, then proceed with therapeutic plasma exchange (TPE)
3. Administer intravenous normal saline to reduce serum viscosity
4. Perform emergent leukocytapheresis to remove circulating B cells producing IgM

Q50. Myeloma cast nephropathy is caused due to aggregation of excessive amounts of __________in distal tubules.

1. Uromodulin
2. Podocin
3. Nephrin
4. KIM-1

Q51. The probability of myeloma cast nephropathy increases with serum level of Free Light Chains (FLC) more than......

1. 1000 mg/L
2. 500md/L
3. 100mg/L
4. 200mg/L

ANSWERS

Q1. Ans(4) Q2. Ans(3) Q3. Ans(4) Q4. Ans(2)

Q5. Ans(3)*[Preferably within 4–8 hours, according to British TTP guidelines.]*

Q6. Ans(4) Q7. Ans(1) Q8. Ans(4) Q9. Ans(4) Q10. Ans(1) Q11. Ans(4)

Q12. Ans(4) Q13. Ans(2) Q14. Ans(2) Q15. Ans(4) Q16. Ans(4) Q17. Ans(4)

Q18. Ans(4) Q19. Ans(4) Q20. Ans(4) Q21. Ans(3) Q22. Ans(4) Q23. Ans(4)

Q24. Ans(4) Q25. Ans(4) Q26. Ans(4) Q27. Ans(2) Q28. Ans(4) Q29. Ans(4)

Q30. Ans(1) Q31. Ans(3) Q32. Ans(1)

Q33. Ans(2& 4)*[FFP is the preferred fluid supplement in TTP and 50.75 ml of 10% calcium gluconate IV is required over the TPE session]*

Q34. Ans(1,3) Q35. Ans(3) Q36. Ans(3) Q37. Ans(2) Q38. Ans(3) Q39. Ans(3)

Q40. Ans(3) Q41. Ans(4) Q42. Ans(4) Q43. Ans(2) Q44. Ans(4) Q45. Ans(4)

Q46. Ans(4) Q47. Ans(4) Q48. Ans(4) Q49. Ans(1)

Q50. Ans(1)*[Uromodulin is otherwise known as Tamm Horsfall proteins. They accumulate in distal tubule causing intratubular obstruction of the lumen of the distal nephron.]*

Q51. Ans(**1**)*[The probability of cast nephropathy increases with the serum level of Free Light Chains(FLC) >1000 mg/L and the amount of its urinary excretion. It rarely occurs at a serum FLC concentration of <500 mg/L.]*

REFERENCES

1. Rubinstein MA, Kagan BM, MacGillivray MH, et al. Unusual remission in a case ofthrombotic thrombocytopenic purpura syndrome following fresh blood exchangetransfusions. Ann Intern Med. 1959;51:1409–19.
2. Bukowski RM, King JW, Hewlett JS. Plasmapheresis in the treatment of thromboticthrombocytopenic purpura. Blood. 1977;50(3):413–7.
3. Bukowski RM, Hewlett JS, Harris JW, et al. Exchange transfusions in the treatment ofthrombotic thrombocytopenic purpura. Semin Hematol. 1976;13(3):219–32.
4. Guidelines on the diagnosis and management of thrombotic thrombocytopenic purpura andother thrombotic microangiopathies. Marie Scully, Beverley J Hunt, Sylvia Benjamin, RiLiesner, Peter Rose, Flora Peyvandi, Betty Cheung, Samuel J MachinBritish Journal ofHaematology 2012; 158 (3):323-335
5. Pathophysiology of thrombotic thrombocytopenic purpura. Tsai HM. Int J Hematol.2010;91:1–19.
6. Thrombotic thrombocytopenic purpura. Joly BS, Coppo P, Veyradier A. Blood.2017;129:2836–2846.
7. Assiri M, AlMalki A, AlHunif B, AlMofareh M. Congenital Thrombotic ThrombocytopenicPurpura: A Rare Cause of Recurrent Thrombocytopenia and Anemia. Cureus. 2023 Sep10;15(9):e44988.
8. ISTH guidelines for treatment of thrombotic thrombocytopenic purpura. Zheng XL, VeselySK, Cataland SR, et al. J Thromb Haemost. 2020;18:2496–2502.
9. Furlan M, Robles R, Galbusera M, Remuzzi G, Kyrle PA, Brenner B, et al. Von willebrandfactor-cleaving protease in thrombotic thrombocytopenic purpura and the hemolytic-uremicsyndrome. N Engl J Med. (1998) 339:1578–84.
10. Pathophysiology of thrombotic thrombocytopenic purpura. Tsai HM. Int J Hematol.2010;91:1–19.
11. Thrombotic thrombocytopenic purpura. Joly BS, Coppo P, Veyradier A. Blood.2017;129:2836–2846.
12. Lee C-H, Huang Y-C, Li S-S, Hsu Y-T, Chen Y-P and Chen T-Y(2022) Application of PLASMIC Scorein Risk Prediction of ThromboticThrombocytopenic Purpura:Real-WorldExperience Froma Tertiary Medical Center in Taiwan. Front. Med. 9:893273.
13. Sutton R, Will A, Kuruvilla M, Victor S. Thrombotic, thrombocytopenic purpura (ADAMTS-13 deficiency): a rare neonatal presentation. Case Reports in Perinatal Medicine. 2015;4(1):73-75.
14. Thrombotic Thrombocytopenic Purpura (TTP) Treatment & ManagementUpdated: Apr 08,2025 Author: Theodore Wun, MD, FACP; Chief Editor: Srikanth Nagalla, MD, MS, FACP more…
15. Lünemann JD, Nimmerjahn F, Dalakas MC. Intravenous immunoglobulinin neurology—modeof action and clinical efficacy. Nat Rev Neurol. 2015;11(2):80–9.
16. Schmidt RE, Budde U, Schäfer G, Stroehmann I. High-doseintravenous gammaglobulin foridiopathic thrombocytopenic purpura. Lancet. 1981;2(8244):475–6.
17. AroraN., Procedures and Protocols in the Neurocritical Care Unit, Switzerland:Springer Nature; 2022.
18. Noiri E. and Hanafusa N., The Concise Manual of Apheresis Therapy. Tokyo: Springer Japan;2014
19. Cid, J., Pérez-Valencia, A. I., Torrente, M. Á., Ávarez-Larrán, A., Díaz-Ricart, M., Esteve, J., & Lozano, M. (2021). Successful management of three patients with autoimmune thromboticthrombocytopenic purpura with paradigm-changing therapy: Caplacizumab, steroids, plasmaexchange, rituximab, and intravenous immunoglobulins (CASPERI). Transfusion andApheresis Science, 60(1), 103011.
20. Zheng XL, Vesely SK, Cataland SR, Coppo P, Geldziler B, Iorio A, et al. Isthguidelines for treatment of thrombotic thrombocytopenic purpura. J Thromb Haemost. (2020) 18:2496–502.
21. Sayani FA, Abrams CS. How I treat refractory thrombotic thrombocytopenic purpura. Blood. 2015; 125:3860–7.
22. Wang, J., Cheng, F., Niu, Y., Yan, L., Li, J., Tan, B., & Qin, L. Therapeutic plasma exchange-free treatment for first-episode TTP: A systematic review. Transfusion and Apheresis Science, 2023;62(3), 103661.
23. Murphy MF, Roberts DJ, Mark H, Yazer NM, editors. Practical Transfusion Medicine Sixth Edition. Hoboken, NJ: John Wiley & Sons, Inc; 2022.
24. Coppo P, Schwarzinger M, Buffet M, Wynckel A, Clabault K, Presne C, et al. Predictivefeatures of severe acquired ADAMTS13 deficiency in idiopathic thromboticmicroangiopathies: the French TMA reference center experience. PLoS One. (2010)5:e10208.
25. Bendapudi, P. K., Li, A., Hamdan, A., Fry, A. M., Uhl, L., Marques, M., Kaufman, R., Stowell, C. P., Dzik, W. S., & Makar, R. S. (2014). Derivation and Prospective Validation of aPredictive Score for the Rapid Diagnosis of Thrombotic Thrombocytopenic Purpura: ThePlasmic Score. Blood, 124(21), 231.
26. Kornblith LZ, Moore HB, Cohen MJ. Trauma-induced coagulopathy: the past, present, andfuture. J Thromb Haemost2019;17(6):852–62
27. O'Leary JG, Greenberg CS, Patton HM, Caldwell SH. AGA clinical practice update:coagulation in cirrhosis. Gastroenterology 2019;157(1):34–43 e1
28. Sukumar S, Lammle B, Cataland SR. Thrombotic thrombocytopenicpurpura:pathophysiology, diagnosis, andmanagement. J Clin Med 2021;10(3):536.

29. Coelho, D. P., Marques, B. A., Roque, A., Carda, J. P., Martinho, P., Fidalgo, T., & Ribeiro, M. L. Comparative Analysis of Clinical Prediction Scores in Acquired ThromboticThrombocytopenic Purpura: The Superiority of Plasmic Score. Blood,2020; 136, 11-12.
30. Zheng XL, Vesely SK, Cataland SR, et al. ISTH guidelines for the diagnosis of thromboticthrombocytopenic purpura. J Thromb Haemost. 2020;18:2486–2495.
31. Li M, Cardigan R, Part S. Practice in Blood Centres and Hospitals Chapter 24:Production and Storage of Blood Components. Blood Centres and Hospitals Chapter. 2022;
32. Pham HP, DePalma H, Williams LA III. Transfusion medicine, haemostasis, apheresis reviewquestions and case studies pretest 1. In: Transfusion Medicine, Apheresis, and Hemostasis.2018. p. 2.
33. Jackups R. Ronald Jackups, MD, PhD — Assistant Professor at Washington University in St. Louis [Internet]. Transfusion News. Available from: https://transfusionnews.com/path-questions/ [cited 2025 Dec 02].
34. Singh A. K. *Core Concepts in Dialysis and Continuous Therapies.* Switzerland:Springer:2016
35. Cooling L, Sherbeck J. Ethylene oxide-type hypersensitivity reactions in G-CSF mobilized, peripheral blood hematopoietic progenitor cell donors and review. J Clin Apher. 2023;38(4):427-436.
36. Adamski J, Ipe TS, Kinard T. Therapeutic and donor apheresis. In: Pham HP, Williams LAIII, editors. Transfusion Medicine, Apheresis, and Hemostasis: Review Questions and Case Studies. 1st ed. London (UK): Academic Press; 2017. p. 327–352.
37. McLeod BC, Szczepiorkowski ZM, Weinstein R, Winters JL, editors. Apheresis: Principles and Practice.3rd ed. Bethesda, MD: AABB; 2010.
38. Sathi BK, Yoshida Y, Weaver MR, Nolan LS, Gruner B, Balasa V, Altes T, Leiva-Salinas C. Unusually High Prevalence of Stroke and Cerebral Vasculopathy in Hemoglobin SC Disease: A Retrospective Single Institution Study. Acta Haematol. 2022;145(2):160-169
39. Connelly-Smith L, Alquist CR, Aqui NA, et al. Guidelines on the Use of Therapeutic Apheresis in Clinical Practice – Evidence-Based Approach from the Writing Committee of the American Society for Apheresis: The Ninth Special Issue. J Clin Apher. 2023; 38(2): 77-278
40. Bain B. Other significant haemoglobinopathies Haemoglobinopathy Diagnosis, 2020:261-324
41. Stubbs LA, Price M, Noland D, Fuchs J, Filkins L, McElvania E, Luu HS, Sebert M, Waters A, Hsiang MS. Transfusion-Transmitted Malaria: Two Pediatric Cases From the United States and Their Relevance in an Increasingly Globalized World. J Pediatric Infect Dis Soc.2021 Dec 31;10(12):1092-1095.
42. Anand Padmanabhan, et al. Guidelines on the use of therapeutic apheresis in clinical practice-evidence-based approach from the writing committee of the American Society for Apheresis. J Clin Apher. 2019; 34:171-354
43. Schwartz J, Padmanabhan A, Aqui N, Balogun RA, Connelly-Smith L, Delaney M, et al. Guidelines on the use of therapeutic apheresis in clinical practice-evidence-based approachfrom the writing Committee of the American Society for apheresis: The seventh SpecialIssue: Therapeutic apheresis-guidelines 2016. J Clin Apher [Internet]. 2016;31(3):149–62.
44. Hemoglobin Screening/Iron Management [monograph on the internet]. Available from:https://www.aabb.org/regulatory-and-advocacy/regulatory-affairs/regulatory-for-blood/donor-safety-screening-and-testing/hemoglobin-screening-iron-management

THERAPEUTIC PLASMA EXCHANGE (TPE) IN LIVER DISEASES AND TRANSPLANT, PANCREAS DISEASES

Dr. Haripriya , Dr. Swapna and Dr. Priyanka

Q1. Which among the following is true in Transplantation?

1. Thomas Earl Starzl performed the first liver transplant and is known as the Father of Modern Transplantation
2. Thomas Earl Starzl performed the world's first liver transplant in Bennie Solis a child at Denver on March 1, 1963
3. Starzl performed baboon-to-human liver xenotransplantation in 1992 and this patient lived 72 days (a milestone for future generations)
4. All of the above

Q2. The MELD Score includes all except:

1. INR
2. Creatinine
3. Bilirubin
4. Serum Sodium

Q3. Which of the following is false in MELD Score?

1. *Malinchoc* along with his coworkers from the Mayo Clinic at Rochester indicated a mathematical model for predicting the result of elective placement of transjugular porto-systemic shunt in patients with cirrhosis and portal hypertension, named the Mayo End-stage Liver Disease (MELD) in 2000
2. The MELD score is *predictive* of survival and is helpful in prioritizing patients with *chronic liver disease* for orthotopic liver transplantation
3. The score also evaluates the prognosis for *fulminant hepatic failure*
4. None of the above

Q4. Which of the following are the disadvantages of MELD score?

1. There is *interlaboratory variation* in measurement of Bilirubin, INR and creatinine
2. It *under estimates* the conditions as malnutrition, portal hypertension and hyponatremia
3. The MELD score is computed by a single measurement of laboratory parameters and hence *it is not a time-dependent model*
4. All of the above

Q5. All of the following are true regarding the Therapeutic apheresis in Liver diseases/transplant except:

1. *Liver transplantation* is indicated for fulminant hepatitis, liver cirrhosis, hepatic cell carcinoma
2. Apheresis as artificial liver support (ALS) plays an important role as a *bridging therapy*
3. Removal of the *albumin bound toxins by means of apheresis (MARS and Prometheus)* is aimed in liver failure
4. None of the above

Q6. Which among the following is a biological/cell based extracorporeal liver support system?

1. Molecular adsorbent recirculating system (MARS)
2. Single pass albumin dialysis (SPAD)
3. Fractionated plasma separation and adsorption (PROMETHEUS)
4. Extracorporeal liver assist device (ELAD)

Q7. All of the following are true in Fulminant Hepatitis except:

1. Fulminant hepatitis is defined if *hepatic coma* (grade II) sets within 8 weeks after the onset and *prothrombin time is below 40%*
2. Hemodiafiltration (HDF) is performed to remove molecules that are not sufficiently removed by PE and which otherwise can cause coma
3. HDF is used either *intermittently or continuously*
4. None of the above

Q8. Which of the following liver conditions are treated by apheresis

1. Acute fatty liver of pregnancy
2. Reye's syndrome
3. Acute Liver Failure
4. All of the above

Q9. Which of the following is true regarding the side effects of Therapeutic apheresis in Liver diseases?

1. The side effects of *plasma exchange* include hypernatremia, metabolic alkalosis, and acute lung oedema due to rapid colloid osmotic pressure enhancement
2. The side effects of *hemodiafiltration* include metabolic acidosis caused by the use of lactate- or acetic acid-based buffers
3. The *metabolism* of acetate and lactate are remarkably reduced in *severe liver failure*
4. All of the above

Q10. Which of the following is true regarding Extracorporeal Liver Systems devices (ECLS)?

1. Extracorporeal Liver Systems devices is separated into two broad categories: *artificial* (A-ECLS) and *bioartificial* ECLS (B-ECLS)
2. A-ECLS devices use endogenous or exogenous *albumin* molecules to bind and scavenge hepatotoxins followed by membrane-based filtration
3. B-ECLS devices use a *cell-based* approach as part of a bioactive system to support hepatic synthetic function and detoxification capacity
4. All of the above

Q11. Which among the following is false regarding the ECLS devices?

1. In Prometheus - A 250-kDa albumin-permeable filter is used to fractionate and separate circulating plasma from the blood
2. The separated plasma is purified through an anion-exchange column and passed through a CRRT circuit before being returned to the patient (Fractionated plasma separation and adsorption device)
3. ECLS can show improvements in serum bilirubin , bile acids and urea levels
4. None of the above

Q12. Which of the following is true regarding treatment of Acute Liver Failure or Acute on Chronic Liver Failure?

1. *Earlier stages* of ALF or ACLF can be treated with PLEX(Plasma Exchange)
2. The treatment with PLEX helps to retard progression of liver failure and helps recovery of liver functions in the native liver
3. In the *later stages* of ALF or ACLF, emergency liver transplantation is the ideal treatment
4. All of the above

Q13. Which of the following is false regarding treatment of ALF or ACLF?

1. The lower blood flow rates during PLEX can result in *lesser hemodynamic fluctuations* in the liver failure patient
2. Patients with ALF or ACLF with *no extra-hepatic organ dysfunction* are *ideal candidates* for PLEX compared to patients with multi-organ failure
3. Liver failure patients who are *not on mechanical ventilation* can tolerate *low-volume PLEX* with the minimal risk of transfusion-related lung complications
4. None of the above

Q14. Which of the following is true regarding PLEX for Hepatitis in India?

1. There are large number of cases during outbreaks of *hepatitis A or E or toxic hepatitis* due to the rodenticide (suicidal agent) ingestion and PLEX is preferred compared to emergency liver transplantation
2. The government of Tamil Nadu has arranged *a triaging system* in each district of Tamil Nadu for identification of patients with rodenticidal hepatotoxicity and provision of PLEX
3. The government of Kerala has encouraged the use of *centrifugal low-volume* PLEX to treat patients with severe acute hepatitis A
4. All of the above

Q15. Which of the following statements are FALSE about Wilson's disease?

1. It is an *autosomal recessive* disease caused by homozygous mutation in ATP7B gene
2. It presents with *DAT negative* haemolytic anaemia
3. TPE is used as *bridge* to transplant in patients with fulminant hepatic failure with *Category I indication and Grade 2C recommendation*
4. TPE is beneficial for rapid removal of significant amounts of copper from the circulation, *an average of 20 mg per TPE treatment*

Q16. All the following statements about erythropoietic protoporphyria (EPP) are true EXCEPT:

1. EPP is an *autosomal recessive disorder* characterised by decreased activity of mitochondrial ferro chelatase
2. Pathogenesis is the accumulation of *metal free protoporphyrin IX*
3. TPE and red cell exchange act as *bridge* to orthotropic liver transplant and/or HSCT
4. RBC exchange *decreases the protoporphyrin levels* in RBC as well as plasma

Q17. The Prometheus (Fractionated Plasma Separation and Adsorption, FPSA) system differs from MARS primarily by:

1. Not using any adsorbent columns
2. Using FFP replacement
3. Direct filtration of albumin through a high-flux filter
4. Removing only water-soluble toxins

Q18. SPAD (Single Pass Albumin Dialysis) differs from MARS in which way?

1. SPAD uses non-regenerated albumin dialysate
2. SPAD has a recirculating albumin circuit
3. SPAD removes fewer albumin-bound toxins
4. SPAD requires separate adsorbent columns

Q19. Which among the following is FALSE about bioartificial liver support devices?

1. Plasma is run through hollow fibre dialysis
2. Contains human hepatoblastoma cell lines or porcine hepatocytes
3. Have better detoxifying capacity than nonbiological artificial liver support systems
4. Have functions of liver such as albumin synthesis

Q20. Find the false statement about Extracorporeal liver assist device (ELAD):

1. Uses porcine hepatocytes
2. Cells are localized in the extra capillary space of a modified dialysis cartridge
3. Cartridges have a membrane cut-off of 70 kDa to prevent the loss of immunoglobulins and blood cells
4. Mimics synthetic and regulatory functions of liver

Q21. Identify the device shown in the Fig VII-1.

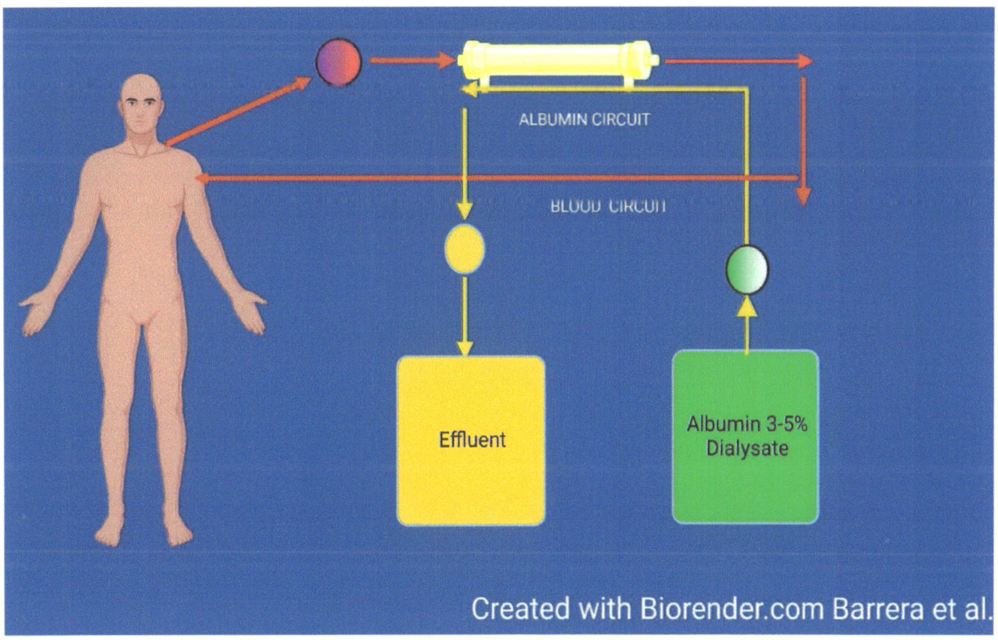

Fig VII-1: Adapted from Villanueva et al.(26) 2023 CCBY(4.0)

1. Molecular adsorbent recirculating system (MARS)
2. Single pass albumin dialysis (SPAD)
3. Fractionated plasma separation and adsorption (PROMETHEUS)
4. Extracorporeal liver assist device (ELAD)

Q22. Identify the device shown in the Fig VII-2.

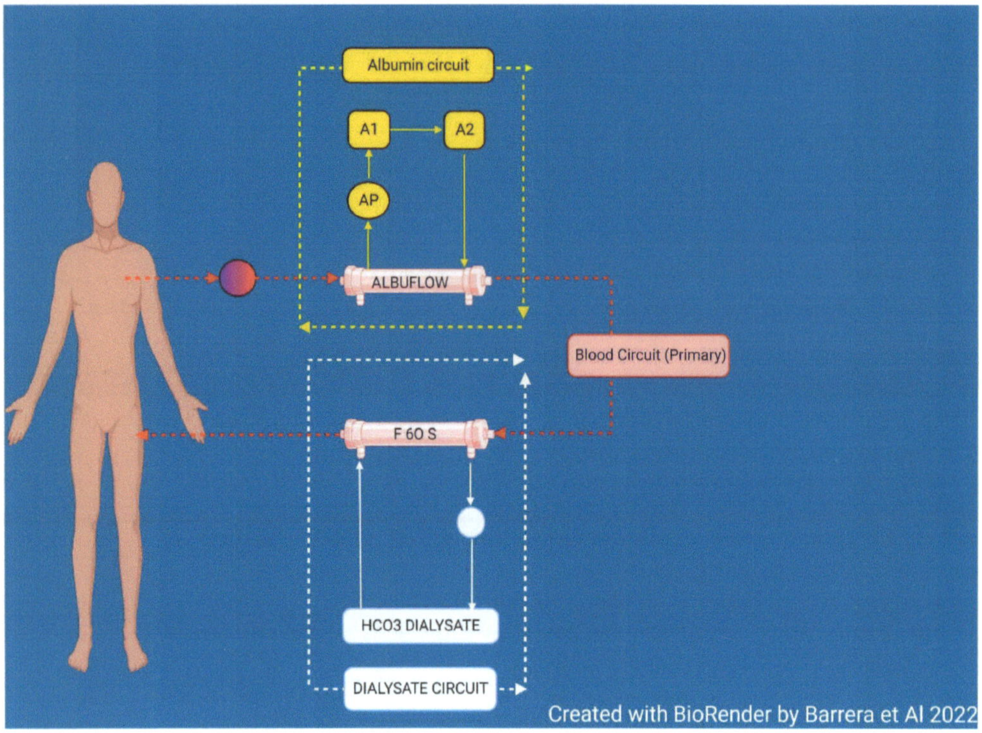

Fig VII-2: Adapted from Villanueva et al.(26) 2023 CCBY(4.0)

1. Molecular adsorbent recirculating system (MARS)
2. Single pass albumin dialysis (SPAD)
3. Fractionated plasma separation and adsorption (PROMETHEUS)
4. Extracorporeal liver assist device (ELAD)

Q23. Which statement about TPE in acute liver failure is TRUE?

1. Contraindicated before transplant
2. Reduces risk of cerebral oedema
3. Worsens coagulopathy
4. Removes albumin-bound toxins better than MARS

Q24. Which statement regarding clinical outcomes of MARS therapy in acute-on-chronic liver failure (ACLF) is supported by evidence in the RELIEF trial?

1. MARS consistently improves overall survival in ACLF
2. MARS improves biochemical parameters but not survival
3. MARS worsens hepatic encephalopathy
4. MARS is contraindicated in renal failure

Q25. Which statement about bioartificial liver (BAL) devices is TRUE?

1. They contain living hepatocytes that provide metabolic support
2. They only work through adsorption
3. They are widely used clinically
4. BAL devices remove toxins only via dialysis

Q26. According to the ASFA 2023 Ninth Special Issue, which therapeutic apheresis procedure is recommended as a Category I indication in acute liver failure?

1. Therapeutic plasma exchange
2. High-volume therapeutic plasma exchange (HV-TPE)
3. CRRT
4. Leukocytapheresis

Q27. Which of the following best defines "high-volume" plasma exchange in acute liver failure?

1. Exchange of 2 plasma volumes per session
2. Exchange of 2–3 litres of plasma
3. Exchange of 8–12 litres
4. Continuous low-volume plasma filtration

Q28. When is the ideal time to reassess laboratory parameters to determine biochemical response in a patient undergoing daily TPE for acute liver failure?

1. Immediately at the completion of each TPE session
2. 12–24 hours after TPE, preferably just before the next exchange
3. After completion of the entire planned course of TPE
4. Six hours after initiation of TPE

Q29. In acute liver failure, HV-TPE is most appropriately used as:

1. Definitive curative therapy
2. Alternative to liver transplantation
3. Bridge to liver transplantation or spontaneous recovery
4. Treatment for chronic liver disease

Q30. Which of the following liver diseases is a retired category IV indication as per ASFA 2023?

1. HELLP syndrome
2. Erythropoeitic protoporphyria liver disease
3. Desensitisation in ABOi liver transplant
4. Wilson's disease

Q31. Which of the following is true regarding therapeutic plasma exchange in Pancreatitis?

1. Patients with severe hypertriglyceridemia (HTG) ie triglyceride levels greater than 1000 mg/dL responded well to plasmapheresis
2. Severe hypertriglyceridemia is responsible for about 1-4% of acute pancreatitis cases
3. TheAmerican Society for Apheresis› guidelines, classified HTGAP (hypertriglyceridemia Acute Pancreatitis) as a Category III indication in case of severe patients and for relapse prevention
4. All of the above

Q32. Which of the following is false regarding therapeutic plasma exchange in Pancreatitis?

1. The first use of plasmapheresis in the treatment of HTG-AP was in 1978 by Betteridge et al.
2. The removal of active enzymes, triglycerides and inflammatory plasma mediators, along with the supplementation of apolipoproteins, free fatty acids, and lipoprotein lipase from a healthy donor, are the advantages of plasmapheresis
3. The majority of HTG instances are secondary and are brought on by disorders that influence lipid metabolism, such as diabetes mellitus, excessive alcohol use, hypothyroidism, pregnancy, or certain drugs including tamoxifen, steroids, and estrogen
4. None of the above

ANSWERS

Q1. Ans(4)

Q2. Ans(4)

Q3. Ans(4)

Q4. Ans(4)

Q5. Ans(4)

Q6. Ans(4)

Hepatocytes are absent from non-biological extracorporeal liver support systems. They depend on adsorption and filtration processes. Eliminating circulating toxins is the goal of artificial extracorporeal liver support systems. Hepatocytes from humans or porcine origin are used in biological/bioartificial ECLS to support the liver's synthetic function and enhance liver detoxification.

Nonbiological

- Molecular adsorbent recirculating system (MARS)
- Single pass albumin dialysis (SPAD)
- Fractionated plasma separation and adsorption (PROMETHEUS)
- Therapeutic plasma exchange (TPE)

Biological

- Hepat Assist device
- Extracorporeal liver assist device (ELAD)
- Modular extracorporeal liver support (MELS)
- Bioartificial liver support system (BLSS)
- Amsterdam Medical Center-bioartifical liver (AMC-BAL)

Q7. Ans(4)

Q8. Ans(4)

Q9. Ans(4)

Q10. Ans(4)

Q11. Ans(4)

Q12. Ans(4)

Q13. Ans(4)

Q14. Ans(4)

Q15. Ans(3)

Wilson disease is an autosomal recessive genetic disorder arising from a mutation in the ATP7B gene, encoding a copper transporting ATPase protein. This mutation leads to impaired biliary copper excretion, resulting in copper accumulation in the liver, brain, cornea, and kidney. The presentation of Wilson's range from asymptomatic liver function test (LFT) abnormalities to hepatitis, cirrhosis, and acute liver failure (ALF). The appearance of Kayser-Fleischer and direct antiglobulin test (DAT) negative haemolytic anaemia are common findings. Wilsons is a category I indication with Grade 1A recommendation

Q16. Ans(4)

The rare autosomal recessive condition known as erythropoietic protoporphyria (EPP) is characterised by decreased activity of the heme biosynthesis pathway enzyme mitochondrial ferrochelatase. As a result, blood levels of metal-free PPIX and erythrocyte total protoporphyrin IX (ePPIX) rise.

During acute protoporphyric liver failure, TPE (Category II Grade 2C) aims to lower the plasma's PPIX level. Additionally, TPE stops PPIX from further depositing in the liver. It might help improve pruritus by eliminating bile acids.

RBC exchange (Category II Grade 2C) is considered a viable option to lower plasma protoporphyrin levels because RBCs can act as a source to absorb excess plasma protoporphyrins. In advanced EPP hepatopathy, combination therapy involving TPE and RBC exchange is useful for reducing liver damage and serving as a bridge to OLT and/or HSCT.

Q17. Ans(3)

Q18. Ans(1)

Blood from patients with SPAD passes through a circuit that has a high-flux hollow fibre haemo diafilter, just like in the MARS system. In contrast to MARS, where it is recirculated, the membrane's other side is cleaned by an albumin solution that flows in counter-direction and is discarded after passing through the filter.

Q19. Ans(3)

The bioartifcial liver support systems have less detoxifying capacity compared to non biological systems, the advantage is that they can reproduce liver functions like albumin synthesis. However the difficulty in maintaining the hepatocytes viable is challenging.

Q20. Ans(1)

Porcine hepatocytes are used in Hepat Assist. ELAD uses hepatoblastoma C3A cell line, derived from human hepatoblastoma cell line HepG2. The modified pore size in the cartridge also prevents tumerogenic hepatocytes from crossing.

Q21. Ans(2)

Q22. Ans(3)

Q23. Ans(2)

Q24. Ans(2)

According to the RELIEF trail MARS; produced a benefit in surrogate parameters of organ dysfunction in ACLF. Treatment with MARS was associated with a decrease in serum bilirubin, with a reduction of serum creatinine to less than 1.5 mg/dL, and with a marked improvement of hepatic encephalopathy (decrease of HE from grade II-IV to grade 0-I) in a high proportion of patients. Despite the beneficial effects of the use of MARS in organ support, no improvement in short-term or mid-term transplant-free survival was observed.

Q25. Ans(1)

Q26. Ans(2)

High-volume therapeutic plasma exchange (HV-TPE) is category I indication whereas TPE is Category III indication.

Q27. Ans(3)

Q28. Ans(2)

Considering recirculation form interstitium, the response to TPE is evaluated in sample drawn the following day (≥ 12 hours or more after TPE).

Q29. Ans(3)

HV TPE helps in providing temporary metabolic support giving time for hepatic regeneration. However, liver transplant is the definitive treatment.

Q30. Ans(1)

The diseases / conditions that were category IV indication in the last guideline and did not have any new evidence were designated as retired category IV indication.

Q31. Ans(4)

Q32. Ans(4)

REFERENCES

1. Brenner DA. Thomas E. Starzl: Transplantation pioneer. Proc Natl Acad Sci U S A.2017;114:10808–10809.
2. Busuttil RW. International Liver Transplantation Society 2009 Presidential Address: The Internationalization of Liver Transplantation. Liver Transpl. 2010;16:558–566.
3. Starzl TE, Fung J, Tzakis A, Todo S, Demetris AJ, Marino IR, Doyle H, Zeevi A, Warty V, Michaels M. Baboon-to-human liver transplantation. Lancet. 1993;341:65–71.
4. Malinchoc, M. · Kamath, P.S. · Gordon, F.D. …A model to predict poor survival in patients undergoing transjugular intrahepatic portosystemic shunts *Hepatology.* 2000; 31:864-871
5. Noiri E and Hanafusa N., The Concise Manual of Apheresis Therapy. Tokyo: Springer Japan;2014
6. Dong V, Karvellas CJ. Liver assistive devices in acute liver failure: Current use and future directions. Best Practice & Research Clinical Gastroenterology. 2024; 73:101961.
7. Kandiah PA, Subramanian RM. Extracorporeal devices. Crit Care Clin 2019;35:135-150.
8. Matar, A. J., & Subramanian, R. (2021). Extracorporeal Liver Support: A Bridge to Somewhere. *Clinical Liver Disease*, *18*(6), 274.
9. Luo HT, Liu QM, Tan JJ, et al. Observation on hybrid bioartificial liver support systems in treating chronic severe hepatitis: a study of 60 cases. Zhonghua Gan Zang Bing Za Zhi. 2006;14(3):205–209.
10. Thomas, R., Eapen, C.E. Plasma exchange to treat liver failure: The field expands. *Indian J Gastroenterol* (2025).
11. Alexander V, Rasalam JE, Kumar S, et al. Transfusion-related lung complications are uncommon in non-ventilated liver failure patients undergoing low-volume plasma exchange. Indian J Gastroenterol. 2024;43:1220–2.
12. Satish SP, Narayanasamy K, Sambandam MT, et al. Christian Medical College (CMC) Vellore collaborative group for PLEX to treat liver failure. The "hub and spoke" model: a pathway for urgent plasma exchange to treat patients with rodenticide ingestion induced acute liver failure in Tamil Nadu India. Lancet Reg Health Southeast Asia. 2024;12:100405.
13. https://dhs.kerala.gov.in/wp-content/uploads/2024/06/Plasma-Exchange_Hepatitis-A_SOP.pdf. Accessed 24 January 2025.
14. AABB. *Apheresis: Principles and Practice*. 4th ed. Bethesda (MD): Association for the Advancement of Blood & Biotherapies; 2020.
15. Connelly-Smith L, Alquist CR, Aqui NA, Hofmann JC, Klingel R, Onwuemene OA, Patriquin CJ, Pham HP, Sanchez AP, Schneiderman J, Witt V, Zantek ND, Dunbar NM. Guidelines on the Use of Therapeutic Apheresis in Clinical Practice - Evidence-Based Approach from the Writing Committee of the American Society for Apheresis: The Ninth Special Issue. J Clin Apher. 2023 Apr;38(2):77-278. doi: 10.1002/jca.22043. PMID: 37017433.
16. Rifai K, Ernst T, Kretschmer U, Bahr MJ, Schneider A, Hafer C, Haller H, Manns MP, Fliser D. Prometheus—a new extracorporeal system for the treatment of liver failure. J Hepatol. 2003; 39(6):984-90.
17. Sauer IM, Goetz M, Steffen I, Walter G, Kehr DC, Schwartlander R, Hwang YJ, Pascher A, Gerlach JC, Neuhaus P. In vitro comparison of the molecular adsorbent recirculation system (MARS) and single-pass albumin dialysis (SPAD). Hepatology. 2004; 39(5):1408-14.
18. Ballester MP, Elshabrawi A, Jalan R. Extracorporeal liver support and liver transplantation for acute-on-chronic liver failure. *Liver Int.* 2025;45:e15647.
19. Kumar Mandal A, Garlapati P, Tiongson B, Gayam V. Liver Assist Devices for Liver Failure [Internet]. Liver Pathology. Intech Open; 2021. Available from: http://dx.doi.org/10.5772/intechopen.91287
20. Bañares R, Nevens F, Larsen FS, Jalan R, Albillos A, Dollinger M, Saliba F, Sauerbruch T, Klammt S, Ockenga J, Pares A, Wendon J, Brünnler T, Kramer L, Mathurin P, de la Mata M, Gasbarrini

A, Müllhaupt B, Wilmer A, Laleman W, Eefsen M, Sen S, Zipprich A, Tenorio T, Pavesi M, Schmidt HH, Mitzner S, Williams R, Arroyo V; RELIEF study group. Extracorporeal albumin dialysis with the molecular adsorbent recirculating system in acute-on-chronic liver failure: the RELIEF trial. Hepatology. 2013; 57(3):1153-62.

21. Pless G, Sauer IM. Bioartificial liver: current status. Transplant Proc. 2005; 37(9):3893-5.
22. Fortson MR, Freedman SN, Webster PD., 3rd Clinical assessment of hyperlipidemic pancreatitis. Am J Gastroenterol. 1995;90:2134–9.
23. Click B, Ketchum AM, Turner R, Whitcomb DC, Papachristou GI, Yadav D. The role of apheresis in hypertriglyceridemia-induced acute pancreatitis: A systematic review. Pancreatology. 2015;15:313–20.
24. Betteridge DJ, Bakowski M, Taylor KG, Reckless JP, de Silva SR, Galton DJ. Treatment of severe diabetic hypertriglyceridaemia by plasma exchange. Lancet. 1978;1:1368.
25. Valdivielso P, Ramirez-Bueno A, Ewald N. Current knowledge of hypertriglyceridemic pancreatitis. Eur J Intern Med. 2014;25:689–94.
26. Villanueva VB, Barrera Amoro´ s DA, CastilloEcheverria EI, Budar-Ferna´ ndez LF, SalasNolasco OI, Juncos LA and Rizo-Topete L. Extracorporeal blood purification inpatients with liver failure: Considerations for the low-and-middle income countries of Latin America. Front. Nephrol. 2023; 3:938710.p5,7

Chapter 8

THERAPEUTIC PLASMA EXCHANGE (TPE) IN RENAL DISEASES AND TRANSPLANT

Dr. Haripriya , Dr. Swapna and Dr. Priyanka

Q1. What is the cut off IgG titre to go ahead with ABOi renal transplant?

1. 8
2. 16
3. 32
4. 64

Q2. In an ABOi renal transplant, what is the approximate number of cycles required for reaching the cut off titre of 16 in a patient with baseline titre of 64?

1. 1-2
2. 2-3
3. 3-4
4. >4

Q3. Based on current market process, ABOi kidney transplant Indian Working Group estimated that immunoadsorption becomes more efficient in reducing antibody titres if more than ___ sessions of plasmapheresis is needed

1. 4
2. 5
3. 6
4. 8

Q4. Which of the following statement is true regarding ABOi renal transplant?

1. TPE should be performed at least 1 week after rituximab therapy
2. IVIG use is generally not recommended
3. Post transplant TPE is necessary in case of graft dysfunction and with increase in titres of >1:16 or a 4 fold increase from baseline
4. All of the above

Q5. A 51 year old male who is a known smoker presented with complaints of fever, fatigue, puffiness of face and leg; and cola coloured urine past for 7 days, followed by decreased urine output for couple of days. Laboratory investigations revealed a Creatinine of 5.9 mg/dL, severe metabolic acidosis, hyperkalaemia. Urine analysis demonstrated low grade proteinuria and RBC casts. Serology revealed high titre anti GBM antibodies. Chest × ray was a normal. Which among the following is not an ideal mode of management?

1. Initiate urgent plasma exchange and continue daily or alternate days up to 10 sessions
2. Initiate immunosuppressive therapy with glucocorticoids, rituximab/ cyclophosphamide under antibiotic cover
3. Perform kidney biopsy for confirmation of diagnosis
4. Initiate urgent haemodialysis

Q6. Which of the following is false regarding therapeutic plasma exchange in anti GBM disease with diffuse alveolar haemorrhage?

1. DAH is a Category I indication with grade 1C recommendation
2. The replacement fluid of choice is 5% albumin
3. TPE is to be performed daily with subsequent reduction in frequency based on clinical course
4. None of the above

Q7. Which immunoadsorption column is used in combination with TPE for treatment of recurrent focal segmental glomerulosclerosis?

1. Immunosorb
2. Glycosorb
3. Cytosorb
4. Globaffin

Q8. Which among the following statements about focal segmental glomerulosclerosis is false?

1. 80% of FSGS is idiopathic
2. Immunoadsorption and TPE are category I indications for FSGS recurrent in kidney transplant
3. Lipoprotein apheresis is a category I indication in all types of FSGS
4. None of the above

Q9. A 46-year-old woman is undergoing a course of therapeutic plasma exchange (TPE) for antibody-mediated renal allograft rejection. A renal biopsy performed the previous evening reveals the following laboratory values: PT 15 seconds and fibrinogen 86 mg/dL. To minimize bleeding risk at the biopsy site, plasma is selected as the replacement fluid. Shortly after initiation of the exchange, the patient develops weakness, headache, confusion, and chest discomfort. The procedure is terminated, and a STAT ionized calcium level is obtained, which is 1.21 mmol/L (reference range: 1.10–1.35 mmol/L). The patient is noted to be receiving cyclosporine therapy. Given these findings, which additional metabolic abnormality related to citrate anticoagulation should be most strongly suspected?

1. Hypomagnesemia
2. Hypercalcemia
3. Hyponatremia
4. Hypermagnesemia

Q10. According to the American Society for Apheresis (ASFA) guidelines summarized in the sources, which condition related to renal transplantation is listed as a Category I indication for Therapeutic Plasma Exchange (TPE)?

1. Posttransplant Focal Segmental Glomerulosclerosis (FSGS)
2. Pretransplant desensitization for HLA incompatibility
3. Treatment of posttransplant Antibody-Mediated Rejection (AMR)
4. Pretransplant desensitization for ABO incompatibility

Q11. Which disease presentation is categorized as Category II 2B for Therapeutic Plasma Exchange in the context of renal disease?

1. Dialysis-independent ANCA-associated Rapidly Progressive Glomerulonephritis (RPGN)
2. Typical diarrhoea-associated Haemolytic Uremic Syndrome (HUS)
3. Myeloma kidney (Cast Nephropathy)
4. Lupus Nephritis

Q12. A 42-year-old male is referred with rapidly rising creatinine and haemoptysis. His lab values are significant for creatinine 4.6mg/dl, Hct 25.0, and anti-GBM 118 units/ml. The renal biopsy shows a severe crescentic glomerulonephritis, involving approximately 69% of glomeruli. The diagnosis is anti-GBM disease with renal and lung involvement. He is started on cyclophosphamide and steroids. He weighs 80 kg. What TPE regimen would you prescribe? An aggressive TPE regimen is required here, as the patient could develop end-stage renal disease and/or fatal pulmonary haemorrhage. A typical regimen would be 1.0–1.5 plasma volumes daily for 10–14 days. After this period, further TPE can be prescribed depending on the anti-GBM titre and the clinical status of the patient. Which among the following in the *prescription* for this patient is false?

1. Remove 6.3 L (1.5 plasma volumes is 6.3 L) and replace with 4.0 L of 5% albumin, 2.0 L of normal saline, and 0.3 L of FFP
2. Premedicate with oral calcium and with oral acetaminophen as well as oral diphenhydramine if there is a possibility of allergic reaction to FFP
3. Give 63 ml of 10% calcium gluconate IV over the TPE
4. None of the above

Q13. Which among the following is false regarding sodium levels during apheresis?

1. Hypernatremia is more common than hyponatremia during apheresis
2. Most hypernatremia cases are due to sodium overload caused by the ACD present in FFP
3. The patient's sodium concentration is monitored every few hours during apheresis
4. None of the above

Q14. Which among the following is true regarding electrolytes during apheresis?

1. The sodium concentration in patients with chronic kidney disease or end stage renal disease is controlled with a combination of apheresis therapy and haemodialysis
2. Combining apheresis therapy with haemodialysis prevents the occurrence of metabolic alkalosis
3. Phosphate levels are evaluated prior to therapy in patients treated with both apheresis and haemodialysis as hypophosphatemia is likely to occur
4. All of the above

Q15. Plasma Exchange and Hemo Dialysis is applied in

1. Diseases with renal failure like Goodpasture's syndrome, complement-mediated diseases, and ANCA-positive vasculitis
2. Infestation with Malarial Parasites
3. Myasthenia gravis and Guillain–Barré syndrome
4. All of the above

Q16. Which of the following is true in Catastrophic Antiphospholipid syndrome (CAPS)?

1. In CAPS, the indication for *TPE is category I, grade 2C* according to the American Society for Apheresis (ASFA), last updated in 2023
2. The disease was first described by *S. Greisman in 1991*. The pathology is also called *Asherson syndrome* in honour of the doctor who first introduced the term "CAPS" in 1992
3. *IAPP* (Cellsorba ® with dextran sulfate ligand), *DFPP and TPE* are the available treatment
4. All of the above

Q17. Which of the following is false in case of ABO-incompatible renal transplantation with respect to lowering of iso agglutinins titres?

1. TPE is required to *remove* significant levels of blood group iso-agglutinins
2. In case plasma is required as part of the replacement for a patient undergoing ABO-incompatible transplantation, the *plasma should not contain ABO antibodies* against the donor kidney
3. The role of TPE in *chronic* antibody-mediated rejection remains *undefined*
4. None of the above

Q18. Which of the following is true in incompatible Renal transplantation Desensitisation protocol?

1. Pretransplantation desensitization protocols mostly use TPE for recipients with living donors who have an incompatible crossmatch from donor-specific human leukocyte antigen (HLA) antibodies
2. The number of TPE sessions is influenced by the degree of sensitization and HLA mismatch
3. IVIG/Rituximab is also used for the elimination of circulating anti-HLA antibodies
4. All of the above

Q19. In case of Antibody-mediated Rejection(AMR) in incompatible Renal Transplant; which of the following is true?

1. Despite the use of desensitisation protocols, about *one third* of the highly sensitised individuals develop acute AMR after transplantation
2. Combined DFPP/rituximab significantly decreased Donor Specific Antibodies in AMR kidney-transplant recipients
3. Target antibodies are mainly IgG anti-donor specific HLA antibodies or anti- A or -B IgG, IgM antibodies
4. All of the above

Q20. Which among the following is false in antibody-mediated rejection in renal transplantation?

1. In Antibody-mediated rejection, TPE is also used in combination with Intravenous immunoglobulin)
2. This condition is I/1B ASFA grade/category indication for TPE
3. In the posttransplant setting, TPE is often used (with variable success) to treat early recurrent focal segmental glomerulosclerosis (FSGS)
4. None of the above

Q21. Post-transplant recurrence of FSGS often responds to plasma exchange because it:

1. Removes circulating permeability factors injuring podocytes
2. Restores nephrin expression
3. Improves graft perfusion
4. Reverses glomerular sclerosis

Q22. Which among the following is false in Rapidly Progressinve Glomerulo Nephritis disease?

1. Laboratory tests indicate the presence of autoantibodies (as MPO-ANCA, PR3- ANCA, or anti-GBM antibody) and apheresis is used to remove the antibodies
2. Antibody titres, urinalysis results, and serum creatinine and C-reactive protein (CRP) levels often correlate with disease activity
3. The initial signs and symptoms include fatigue, fever, anorexia, oedema, bubbles in the urine related to proteinuria, haematuria, nausea, and weight loss and extra-renal symptoms include joint pain, muscle pain, haemoptysis, purpura, and melena
4. None of the above

Q23. What is the etiological factor most strongly associated with the development of nephrogenic systemic fibrosis (NSF)?

1. Chronic exposure to iodinated contrast media
2. Administration of gadolinium-based contrast agents in patients with renal failure
3. Long-term corticosteroid therapy
4. Autoimmune connective tissue disease

Q24. Which of the following statements is true about Prospective Observational Survey on the Long-Term Effects of LDL Apheresis on the Drug Resistant Nephrotic Syndrome (POLARIS) study?

1. It is a prospective observational survey on the long-term effect of LDL apheresis on drug-resistant Nephrotic Syndrome (NS)
2. LDL apheresis curtailed proteinuria in nearly half of the patients with NS who failed to respond to primary mode of medication
3. LDL apheresis was scheduled 2 times per week for 3 weeks followed by 6 weekly treatments
4. All of the above

ANSWERS

Q1. Ans(2)
In ABOi renal transplants, assessment of one antibody titre before subjecting patient to antibody removal is recommended. IgG measurement should be used to make clinical decisions whereas IgM measurement is discretionary. Pretransplant IgG antibody titer of ≤ 1:16 should be taken as cut-off for ABOi-renal transplant.

Q2. Ans(2)
Approximately, number of cycles required to reach a target titre of <1:16 in an ABOi renal transplant will be 1–2, 2–3, 3–4, 4–5, 5–6, and >6 for baseline titres of <32, 64, 128, 256, 512, and >512, respectively.

Q3. Ans(1)
The major disadvantage immunoadsorption is the high cost. Hence it is not a preferred method for antibody removal in cases where pretransplant titres are low. The working group estimated that immunoadsorption becomes efficient in cases where more than 4 sessions of TPE is required. Hence it is ideal to use immunoadsorption in cases with pretransplant titres of more than 128.

Q4. Ans(4)

Q5. Ans(1)
Patients with Serum creatine level of more than 5.7 mg/dL and dialysis dependence at time of presentation may not benefit from TPE. The risk vs benefit of TPE is to be evaluated in such cases. When patient develops diffuse alveolar haemorrhage which is rapidly fatal, TPE is preferably initiated.

Q6. Ans(2)
The fluid of choice in case if diffuse alveolar haemorrhage is FFP. FFP is to be used as part or whole of replacement fluid.

Q7. Ans(1)
Some patients with recurrent FSGS have been treated with partial success with a combination of TPE and IA with staphylococcal protein A columns.

Q8. Ans(3)
LA is a category II indication in all types of FSGS. The altered lipid metabolism in nephrotic syndrome causes hypercholesterolemia, which leads to a lipotoxic environment causing podocyte damage- the rationale for LA is to reduce the same.

Q9. Ans(1)

Q10. Ans(3)

Q11. Ans(3)

Q12. Ans(4)
FFP is administered for the renal biopsy and hemoptysis. FFP may also be issued if bleeding is a significant, and more FFP and less normal saline would have been administered.

Even more IV calcium gluconate is needed if the patient was given additional FFP.

Note: had DFPP been performed the prescription would just be to remove 6.3 L of plasma and replace with small volume of 5% albumin (as only a small amount being removed). FFP and/or fibrinogen is administered only according to laboratory evidence of a coagulopathy.

Q13. Ans(4)

Q14. Ans(4)

Q15. Ans(4)

Q16. Ans(4)

Q17. Ans(4)

Q18. Ans(4)

Q19. Ans(4)

Q20. Ans(4)

Q21. Ans(1)

The circulating factors seen in patients with recurrent FSGS increases glomerular permeability. The decreasing plasma concentration of these factors coincides with improvement in proteinuria. TPE is usually started once recurrence is diagnosed. The number of TPE procedures to decrease proteinuria is variable according to studies.

Q22. Ans(4)

Q23. Ans(2)

Nephrogenic systemic fibrosis is a rare and fatal disorder occurring in patients with acute or chronic kidney disease following the administration of gadolinium based contrast agents. ECP/TPE is Category III indication with GRADE 2C recommendation.

Q24. Ans(4)

REFERENCES

1. Montgomery RA, Locke JE, King KE, Segev DL, Warren DS, Kraus ES, *et al.* ABO incompatible renal transplantation: A paradigm ready for broad implementation. Transplantation 2009;87:1246-55
2. Bhalla AK, Kumar BT, Chauhan M, Das P, Gandhi B, Hegde U, *et al.* ABO-incompatible kidncy transplantation: Indian working group recommendations. Indian J Transplant 2019;13:252-8.
3. Connelly-Smith L, Alquist CR, Aqui NA, Hofmann JC, Klingel R, Onwuemene OA, Patriquin CJ, Pham HP, Sanchez AP, Schneiderman J, Witt V, Zantek ND, Dunbar NM. Guidelines on the Use of Therapeutic Apheresis in Clinical Practice - Evidence-Based Approach from the Writing Committee of the American Society for Apheresis: The Ninth Special Issue. J Clin Apher. 2023 Apr;38(2):77-278. doi: 10.1002/jca.22043. PMID: 37017433.
4. Adamski J, Ipe TS, Kinard T. Therapeutic and donor apheresis. In: Pham HP, Williams LA III, editors. *Transfusion Medicine, Apheresis, and Hemostasis: Review Questions and Case Studies*. 1st ed. London (UK): Academic Press; 2017. p. 327–352.
5. McLeod BC, Szczepiorkowski ZM, Weinstein R, Winters JL, editors. Apheresis: Principles and Practice. 3rd ed. Bethesda, MD: AABB; 2010.
6. Singh A.K. *Core Concepts in Dialysis and Continuous Therapies.* Switzerland:Springer:2016
7. Noiri E. and Hanafusa N., The Concise Manual of Apheresis Therapy. Tokyo:Springer Japan;2014
8. Asherson R.A. The catastrophic antiphospholipid syndrome. J. Rheumatol. 1992;19:508–512.
9. Bitsadze V, Yakubova F, Khizroeva J, Lazarchuk A, Salnikova P, Vorobev A, Tretyakova M, Degtyareva N, Grigoreva K, Gashimova N, Kvaratskheliia M, Makatsariya N, Kudryavtseva E, Tomlenova A, Gris JC, Elalamy I, Ay C, Makatsariya A. Catastrophic Antiphospholipid Syndrome. Int J Mol Sci. 2024; 25(1):668.
10. Desensitization in kidney transplantation: Review Jamilya Saparbay1, Mels Assykbayev1, Saitkarim Abdugafarov1, Gulnur Zhakhina1, Janat Spatayev1. Vol. 18. Asan Zhexembayev, Zhuldyz Zhanzakova, Aida Turganbekova, Saniya Abdrakhmanova; Kazakhstan; 2021.
11. Vo AA, Choi J, Cisneros K, et al Benefits of rituximab combined with intravenous immuno-globulin for desensitization in kidney transplant recipients Transplantation. 2014;98(3):312–9
12. Noble, Johan MD1,2; Jouve, Thomas MD, PhD1,2; Malvezzi, Paolo MD1; Rostaing, Lionel MD, PhD1,2,3. Desensitization in Crossmatch-positive Kidney Transplant Candidates. Transplantation 2023;107(2):p 351-360.
13. Naciri Bennani H, Daligault M, Noble J, Bardy B, Motte L, Giovannini D, et al. Treatment of antibody-mediated rejection with double-filtration plasmapheresis, low dose IVIg plus rituximab after kidney transplantation. J Clin Apher [Internet]. 2021;36(4):584–94.
14. Chehade H, Pascual M. The challenge of acute antibody-mediated rejection in kidney transplantation Transplantation., 100 (2016), pp. 264-265
15. Artero ML, Sharma R, Savin VJ, Vincenti F. Plasmapheresis reducesproteinuria and serum capacity to injure glomeruli in patients with recurrent focal glomerulosclerosis. Am J Kidney Dis.1994;23(4):574–81.

16. Muso E, Mune M, Hirano T, Hattori M, Kimura K, Watanabe T, Yokoyama H, Sato H, Uchida S, Wada T, Shoji T, Takemura T, Yuzawa Y, Ogahara S, Sugiyama S, Iino Y, Sakai S, Ogura Y, Yukawa S, Nishizawa Y, Yorioka N, Imai E, Matsuo S, Saito T. A Prospective Observational Survey on the Long-Term Effect of LDL Apheresis on Drug-Resistant Nephrotic Syndrome. Nephron Extra. 2015;5(2):58-66.
17. Ou TY, Chuang CY, Chen CD, Cheng CY. Therapeutic plasma exchange in the treatment of complicated Plasmodium falciparum malaria: A case report. J Clin Apher. 2018; 33(3):419-422.
18. Schaefer, B., Ujszaszi, A., Schaefer, S., Heckert, K. H., Schaefer, F., & Schmitt, C. P. Safety and Efficacy of Tandem Hemodialysis and Plasma Exchange in Children. *Clinical Journal of the American Society of Nephrology*: CJASN, 2014; 9(9), 1563.

Chapter 9

THERAPEUTIC PLASMA EXCHANGE (TPE) AND DRUG INTERACTIONS

Dr. Swapna and Dr. Sunantha

Q1. Which of the following is false?

1. Pharmacodynamics is defined as physiological and biochemical effects of drugs and their mechanism of action at organ system/subcellular/macromolecular levels
2. Pharmacokinetics is defined as movement of the drug in and alteration of the drug by the body; includes absorption, distribution, binding/localization/storage, bio-transformation, and excretion of the drug
3. Pharmacogenomics represents an expanding field within genomic medicine that utilizes a patient's genetic information to assist healthcare professionals in choosing the medications and dosages anticipated to be most effective for each individual patient
4. None of the above

Q2. Which of the following regarding the Volume of distribution is not true?

1. It is expressed as the volume of the substance per body weight (L/kg)
2. Volume of distribution can vastly exceed any physical volume in the body because it is the volume *apparently* necessary to contain the amount of drug *homogeneously* at the concentration found in the blood, plasma, or water
3. Drugs that are completely retained within the vascular compartment have a minimum possible volume of distribution equal to the blood component in which they are distributed
4. None of the above

Q3. Which of the following regarding the Clearance is not true?

1. It is given by the formula; Clearance = Rate of elimination/ Concentration of drug
2. Clearance of a drug is the factor that predicts the rate of elimination in relation to the drug concentration
3. Clearance in first order kinetics is constant
4. Clearance in zero order kinetics is constant

Q4. Which of the following regarding plasma half life is true?

1. The Plasma half-life (t½) of a drug is the time taken for its plasma concentration to be reduced to half of its original value
2. The half life depends on volume of distribution and clearance
3. Most useful in designing drug dosage regimens when the body is considered as a single compartment
4. All of the above

Q5. Which of the following is not true regarding one- compartment model?

1. A one-compartment model is used for drugs which rapidly equilibrate with the tissue compartment
2. The one-compartment model in pharmacokinetics simplifies the body into a single, homogenous unit where a drug distributes instantaneously and is eliminated at a constant rate
3. Drug elimination within the compartment occurs following apparent zero-order kinetics
4. An example for one-compartment model is aminoglycosides

Q6. Which of the following is true regarding two- compartment model?

1. The two-compartment pharmacokinetic model describes the evolution of drug levels in the organism by depicting the body as two pharmacokinetic compartments
2. Once a given drug amount reaches one of the compartments, it distributes throughout it immediately and homogenously
3. When a drug follows a two-compartment model, its concentration in the plasma follows a bi-exponential curve, reflecting two distinct phases
4. All of the above

Q7. Which of the following is true regarding three- compartment model and multi compartment?

1. The net effect of having multiple compartments is that there is an initial fast distribution phase, followed by a slower elimination phase during which the concentration is maintained by redistribution from drug stores in the tissues
2. The three-compartment model has elimination phase alpha, distribution phase beta, terminal phase gamma
3. Elimination t½ = ln2/k; Where ln2 is the natural logarithm of 2 (or 0.693) and *k* is the *elimination rate constant* of the drug, i.e. the fraction of the total amount of drug in the body which is removed per unit time
4. All of the above

Q8. The following are true regarding protein bound drugs except

1. Drugs such as salicylates and disopyramide are extensively bound to plasma albumin
2. The α1-Acid glycoprotein is an important binding protein with binding sites for drugs such as lidocaine and propranolol
3. High plasma protein binding affinity allows drugs to remain in the intravascular compartment
4. High plasma protein binding affinity enhances the production rate of drugs

Q9. Which of the following is not true regarding the role of Albumin and TPE?

1. Albumin is responsible for most nonspecific protein binding of drugs
2. Alzheimer Management by Albumin Replacement ("AMBAR") study investigated the effects of plasmapheresis with albumin replacement in patients with mild-to-moderate Alzheimer's disease (AD)
3. TPE is mostly unaffected by molecular weight or protein binding rate and has the largest range for removal of toxic substances
4. None of the above

Q10. In which phase the drug is most susceptible to TPE?

1. Drug Ingestion phase
2. Drug Distribution phase
3. Drug Elimination phase
4. Any of the above

Q11. Which among the following is false regarding replacement fluids in TPE for Drug intoxication?

1. In a case of drug overdose, the American Society for Apheresis (ASFA) guidelines indicates the use of albumin or fresh-frozen plasma (FFP) based on the specific drug-binding features to help draw the medication/drug into the intravascular space
2. The removal of plasma without albumin replacement can increase the free fraction of drugs after redistribution which decreases the clinical toxicity
3. The use of FFP is beneficial in case of overdose with high α1-acid glycoprotein affinity drugs, such as quinidine
4. The use of 5%Human Albumin Serum is beneficial in case of overdose with high α1-acid glycoprotein affinity drugs, such as quinidine

Q12. Which of the following is not true regarding TPE procedure in Drug Intoxication?

1. TPE is most likely to remove drugs with a very low volume of distribution (<0.2 L/kg)
2. TPE is most likely to remove drugs with high protein binding (>80%)
3. The choice of replacement fluid can also have a clinical effect on drug levels
4. The choice of replacement fluid does not have a clinical effect on free fractions of circulating medications

Q13. All the following drugs are removed during TPE except

1. Mycophenolate
2. Rituximab
3. Cisplatin
4. Tacrolimus

Q14. Which of the following is true regarding the impact of TPE and the removal of drugs?

1. Ampicillin- Moderately affected
2. Ceftriaxone – Not affected
3. Tobramycin- Moderately Affected
4. Ampicillin- Not affected

Q15. Which of the following drug removal is affected by TPE?

1. Cefepime
2. Acylcovir
3. Voriconazole
4. Liposomal Amphotericin B

Q16. Which of the following group of drugs have been significantly impacted by TPE?

1. Antivirals
2. Antiepileptic
3. Antithrombotics
4. Fluoroquinolones

Q17. TPE is effective in elimination of

1. Ethylene dibromide poisoning cases
2. Mercury poisoning cases
3. Diltiazem & Verapamil Intoxications
4. All of the above

Q18. TPE and other extracorporeal methods are effective in drug intoxications caused by

1. Amitriptyline
2. Theophylline
3. Procainamide
4. All of the above

Q19. Hemodialysis is the best treatment for

1. Methanol Toxicosis
2. Ethylene Glycol
3. Ethanol Toxicosis
4. All of the above

Q20. Which among the following is true regarding antiepileptics elimination?

1. Phenytoin, valproic acid, phenobarbital, oxcarbazepine, and carbamazepine all have high protein binding (70% to 90%)
2. These drugs have moderate to high V_D (volume of distribution) ranging from 0.6 to 1.9 L/kg
3. These drugs exhibit poor removal via TPE due to their vast extravascular tissue distribution and significant post procedure rebound
4. All of the above

Q21. Indications for blood purification (extracorporeal techniques) in drug toxicosis include all except

1. The general state gradually worsens despite the standard treatment
2. Brainstem dysfunction (hypotension, hypothermia, respiratory depression etc.)
3. Deep coma with pneumonia or sepsis
4. None of the above

Q22. Which of the following are indications for blood purification in drug toxicosis?

1. Severe organ injury is present that affects the metabolism of the causative agent
2. The metabolic products of the causative agents have toxicity
3. The causative agents may cause delayed organ injury
4. All of the above

Q23. In case of yellow phosphorus poisoning, which of the following is true?

1. TPE is not routinely recommended in the management of yellow phosphorus
2. TPE is recommended only as a 'bridge to liver transplantation'
3. Successful outcome of TPE depends on early detection and management of associated life threatening complications such as hypocalcaemia, hypoglycaemia, hepatic encephalopathy, cerebral oedema and spontaneous bleeding
4. All of the above

Q24. In case of yellow phosphorus poisoning when TPE is performed which of the following is true?

1. Hypoglycaemia settles along with liver enzymes within the first 2 weeks of onset of Acute Liver Failure
2. Bilirubin and prothrombin time take at least 6 weeks to normalise
3. Urea levels are the last to recover
4. All of the above

Q25. Which of the following is false in Paraquat poisoning?

1. Paraquat is a toxic herbicide that impairs renal function; is not significantly protein bound and has a short half-life
2. Its presence in the circulation is prolonged because elimination depends on renal function
3. The total removal by plasmapheresis is reported as nonsignificant in the context of endogenous metabolic clearance
4. None of the above

Q26. Which of the following is true in case of Plasmapheresis for Chemotherapeutic Agents?

1. Plasmapheresis is used for cases of vincristine and cisplatin overdose
2. The reduction in the plasma concentrations of cisplatin is seen with plasmapheresis but there is rebound phenomenon
3. Plasmapheresis is justified because of high protein binding and the absence of recognized therapy
4. All of the above

Q27. Which of the following is false in Plasmapheresis for thyroid hormones?

1. Most reports of plasmapheresis for the removal of thyroid hormones are promising
2. A single exchange procedure will not decrease serum thyroxine levels significantly (as there is rapid rebound of thyroid hormone from the tissues into the plasma)
3. Plasmapheresis and charcoal hemoperfusion are effective in decreasing the duration of thyroxine intoxication
4. None of the above

Q28. Plasmapheresis has demonstrated possible benefit in

1. Natalizumab clearance
2. Amlodipine poisoning
3. When the *type and amount* of the causative toxic substance is unknown
4. All of the above

Q29. Which of the following is false in Amanita poisonings?

1. The lethal dose of amanita toxin is 0.1 mg/kg body weight (severe poisoning can occur with amount as small as 5 to 7 mg of amanita toxin)
2. The amanita toxin is eliminated by the kidneys and often undetectable in the plasma 48 hours after ingestion and swift therapeutic intervention is required to mitigate dangerous complications
3. However, there is no clear evidence to support the use of Plasmapheresis despite a category II indication for plasmapheresis by the American Society for Apheresis (ASFA) guidelines
4. None of the above

ANSWERS

Q1. Ans(4)

Q2. Ans(4)

Q3. Ans(4)

First order kinetics: The rate of elimination is directly proportional to the drug concentration, Clearance remains constant; or a constant fraction of the drug present in the body is eliminated in unit time.

Zero order kinetics: The rate of elimination remains constant irrespective of drug concentration, Clearance decreases with increase in concentration; or a constant amount of the drug is eliminated in unit time.

Q4. Ans(4)

Q5. Ans(3)

Q6. Ans(4)

The dual compartments

Central Compartment: This compartment includes the bloodstream and organs that have a high blood perfusion rate, such as the heart, liver, and kidneys. When a medication is administered intravenously, it immediately enters this compartment. The elimination process, whether through metabolism or excretion, is believed to primarily occur from the central compartment.

Peripheral Compartment: This compartment consists of tissues that have lower blood perfusion, including muscle, adipose tissue, dermis, and connective tissue. It is sometimes referred to as the "tissue compartment." The medication moves into and out of this compartment at a slower rate.

Q7. Ans(4)

Q8. Ans(4)

Q9. Ans(4)

Q10. Ans(2)

Q11. Ans(4)

Q12. Ans(4)

Q13. Ans(4)

Q14. Ans(1)

Q15. Ans(4)

Q16. Ans(3)

Q17. Ans(4)

Q18. Ans(4)

Q19. Ans(4)

Q20. Ans(4)

Q21. Ans(4)

Q22. Ans(4)

Q23. Ans(4)

Q24. Ans(4)

Q25. Ans(4)

Q26. Ans(4)

Q27. Ans(4)

Q28. Ans(4)

Q29. Ans(4)

REFERENCES

1. Holford NHG. Pharmacokinetics and pharmacodynamics: rational dosing and the time course ofdrug action. VanderahVT. Katzung BG. Basic and Clinical Pharmacology. 16th ed. New York:McGraw Hill; 2024.p.42-45.
2. Katzung BG. Basic & Clinical Pharmacology. Pharmacokinetics & Pharmacodynamics: Rational Dosing & the Time Course of Drug Action 14th ed. New York: McGraw-Hill Education; 2018: 37-41.
3. Pharmacokinetics: Metabolism and Excretion of Drugs, Kinetics of Elimination:Tripathi KD. Essentials of Medical Pharmacology. 11th ed. New Delhi: Jaypee Brothers MedicalPublishers; 2023.
4. Talevi A, The ADME Encyclopedia: A Comprehensive Guide on Biopharmacy andPharmacokinetics. Cham: Springer Nature Switzerland AG; 2022.
5. Cheng JE, Hendrickson, Sidhu D, Jd MD. Therapeutic Plasma Exchange and Its Impact on Drug Levels An ACLPS Critical ReviewCaleb W. Vol. 148. MD,1,2 Christopher A. Tormey, MD,1; 2017.
6. Noiri E.and Hanafusa N., The Concise Manual of Apheresis Therapy. Tokyo: Springer Japan;2014
7. Mahmoud SH, Buhler J, Chu E, Chen SA, Human T. Drug Dosing in Patients Undergoing Therapeutic Plasma Exchange. Neurocritical Care. 2020 May 22;34(1):301–11.
8. Schwartz J, Padmanabhan A, Aqui N, Balogun RA, Connelly-Smith L, Delaney M, Dunbar NM, Witt V, Wu Y, Shaz BH. Guidelines on the Use of Therapeutic Apheresis in Clinical Practice-Evidence-Based Approach from the Writing Committee of the American Society for Apheresis: The Seventh Special Issue. J Clin Apher. 2016 Jun;31(3):149-62.

9. Ghannoum M, Roberts DM, Hoffman RS, Ouellet G, Roy L, Decker BS, Bouchard J. A stepwise approach for the management of poisoning with extracorporeal treatments. Semin Dial. 2014; 27(4):362-70.
10. Roberts DM, Buckley NA. Pharmacokinetic considerations in clinical toxicology: clinical applications. Clin Pharmacokinet. 2007;46(11):897-939.
11. Is Antimicrobial Treatment Effective During Therapeutic Plasma Exchange? Investigating the Role of Possible Interactions Łukasz J. Krzych 1,*, Marcelina Czok 2 and Zbigniew Putowski *Pharmaceutics* 2020, *12*, 395;
12. Pahwa, N., Bharani, R., Jain, M., Argal, S., Soni, H., Kosta, S., & Kumar, R. (2013). Therapeutic plasma exchange: An effective treatment in ethylene dibromide poisoning cases. *Journal of Clinical Apheresis*, *28*(5), 374-377.
13. Patel, N., and Bayliss G. P. Developments in extracorporeal therapy for the poisoned patient. Adv. Drug Deliv. Rev.2015; 90:3–11.
14. Dişel, N. R., Akpınar, A. A., Sebe, A., Karakoç, E., Sürer, S., Turhan, F. T., and Matyar, S. Therapeutic plasma exchange in poisoning: 8 years' experience of a university hospital. Am. J. Emerg. Med. 2015;33:1391–1395.
15. Lavergne, V., Nolin T. D., Hoffman R. S., et al. The EXTRIP (EXtracorporeal TReatments in poisoning) workgroup: guideline methodology. Clin. Toxicol. 2012; 50:403–413.
16. Sari, I., Turkcuer I., Erurker T., Serinken M., Seyit M., and Keskin A.. Therapeutic plasma exchange in amitriptyline intoxication: case report and review of the literature. Transfus. Apher. Sci. 2011;45:183–185.
17. Ibrahim RB, Balogun RA. Medications in patients treated with therapeutic plasma exchange: prescription dosage, timing, and drug overdose. Semin Dial. 2012; 25(2):176-89.
18. Modified Japanese Society for Clinical Toxicology Guidelines(http://journalsonline.tandf.co.uk/media/f83gxpxyvj02my13xxb0/contributions/t/g/c/q/tgcq8hk3u9xn0e6r.pdf)
19. Mathew, J., Gnanaraj, J., Basavarajegowda, A., & Venkateswaran, R. Plasmapheresis in lethal yellow phosphorus poisoning: A scope for recovery. *BMJ Case Reports*,2021; *14*(4), e239676.
20. C Ronco, R Bellomo, Kellum JA, Zaccaria Ricci. Critical care nephrology. 3rd edition. Plasmapheresis in Acute Intoxication and Poisoning *François Madore and Josée Bouchard* Philadelphia, Pa: Elsevier; 2019.*p.595-600*
21. Edison, D. C., Philip, J., Mallhi, R., Basnotra, R., Pynadath, V., & Sane, K. Severe amlodipine toxicity: A medical dilemma managed with therapeutic plasma exchange. *Transfusion and Apheresis Science*,2024; *63*(4), 103958.
22. Shemin D, Briggs D, Greenan M. Complications of therapeutic plasma exchange: a prospective study of 1,727 procedures. J Clin Apher. 2007;22(5):270–6.
23. Lu J, Zhang L, Xia C, Tao Y. Complications of therapeutic plasma exchange: a retrospective study of 1201 procedures in 435 children. Medicine (Baltimore). 2019;98(50):e18308.

Chapter 10

THERAPEUTIC PLASMA EXCHANGE IN MISCELLANEOUS CONDITIONS

Dr. Swapna and Dr. Haripriya

Q1. In case of Steven–Johnson Syndrome and Toxic Epidermal Necrolysis, which of the following is true?

1. The target substance removed is proinflammatory cytokines such as TNF- α and IFN- γ
2. Soluble Fas ligand is also one of the target substances
3. PE or DFPP is proposed during the early stages of the disease if glucocorticoids are ineffective
4. All of the above

Q2. In case of Pemphigus and Pemphigoid, which of the following is true?

1. Removal of antibodies by apheresis is not recommended
2. Apheresis helps removal of specific autoantibodies of IgG class against adhesion molecules in skin tissues
3. Apheresis helps removal of specific autoantibodies of IgA class against adhesion molecules in skin tissues
4. Apheresis helps removal of smooth muscle antibodies

Q3. For the treatment of Pemphigus and Pemphigoid; which of the following is true?

1. Pemphigus is an autoimmune bullous disease where desmoglein (Dsg), an epidermal cell adhesion molecule, is aimed by autoantibodies
2. Apheresis is performed to remove IgG autoantibodies, in *severe or refractory* pemphigus and pemphigoid
3. Apheresis is recommended from an early stage as a life-saving procedure in case of serious and life-threatening toxic epidermal necrosis
4. All of the above

Q4. IgA nephropathy (Berger'disease) crescentic and chronic progressive types are indications for

1. TPE III and grade 2B
2. TPE III and Grade 2C
3. TPE III and grade 2B and 2C respectively
4. TPE III and grade 2C and 2B respectively

Q5. Which among the following statements is false regarding TPE in IgA nephropathy?

1. Removes plasma IgA-IgG complexes and complement products
2. Fixed course therapy of 6 to 9 sessions over 21 days is recommended
3. Creatinine is not usually monitored for determining the response
4. TPE is category III indication

Q6. Which of the following is false in Rheumatoid Arthritis?

1. Therapeutic apheresis is used for the treatment of rheumatoid arthritis which does not respond to pharmacologic treatments
2. Therapeutic apheresis is performed to remove infiltrating activated T cells, B cells, neutrophils, and monocytes in patients with rheumatoid arthritis
3. Filtration leukocytapheresis (LCAP) has dose dependent effects
4. Therapeutic apheresis is not used in addition to medical management (glucocorticoids or immunosuppressants) in case of Malignant Rheumatoid arthritis

Q7. Which of the following is false in Systemic Lupus Erythematosus?

1. Therapeutic apheresis therapy is used for the treatment of systemic lupus erythematosus (SLE) that is associated with severe organ damage despite treatment with glucocorticoids or immunosuppressive agents
2. Therapeutic apheresis removes immune complexes and autoantibodies [anti-double-strand (ds) DNA antibodies etc.] in these patients
3. Plasma exchange (PE), double filtration plasmapheresis (DFPP), cryofiltration, or immunoadsorption plasmapheresis (IAPP) are chosen based on the disease status of each patient
4. None of the above

Q8. Effect of TPE in patients with which of the following was studied in the MEPEX trial?

1. Recurrent FSGS
2. ANCA vasculitis
3. Myeloma cast nephropathy
4. IgA nephropathy

Q9. Which of the following is false in ANCA-Associated Vasculitis?

1. Therapeutic apheresis is performed for patients with ANCA-associated vasculitis that is resistant to a combination of glucocorticoids and immunosuppressive agents
2. Therapeutic apheresis is performed for patients with ANCA-associated vasculitis when it is complicated with rapidly progressive glomerulonephritis (RPGN) or pulmonary bleeding
3. Plasma Exchange removes autoantibodies (e.g., ANCA, anti-LAMP2 antibodies, anti plasminogen)
4. None of the above

Q10. Which of the following is true in the treatment of ANCA-Associated Vasculitis (AAV)?

1. The targets for removal are activated leukocytes, activated macrophages, complement, adhesion molecules, cytokines, and chemokines apart from autoantibodies
2. PE is preferentially used and is initially performed two or three times a week
3. The treatment interval for PE is prolonged according to the clinical response and DFPP is used for maintenance therapy
4. All of the above

Q11. Which of the following is false in Neonatal Lupus?

1. Neonatal lupus is caused by transplacental passage of maternal anti-SS-A and/or anti-SS-B IgG antibodies and they are responsible for congenital heart block in infants (2% is the frequency)
2. The maternal IgG antibodies pass into the fetal circulation via active placental transfer and result in complete atrioventricular block, often detected between 18 and 24 weeks gestation
3. To prevent fetal conduction failure, pregnant women with highly elevated levels of SSA-antibodies and/or a positive history of clinical complications are treated with IAPP
4. None of the above

Q12. P and P k antigens present on the surface of erythrocytes are also expressed in the chorion. Anti-PP 1 P k antibodies detected in the circulation of mothers lacking P, P 1, or P k antigens (small p type) blood group antigens can disrupt placental function, potentially leading to intrauterine growth retardation or intrauterine fetal loss. When a patient early in gestation reports, which of the following is true?

1. In early gestation, till the time fetal blood transfusion is performed safely, apheresis is used
2. The apheresis treatment is continued until late pregnancy, with a decreased frequency
3. Apheresis is contraindicated in pregnancy
4. (1 &2)

Q13. Which of the following is true in pregnancy due to Rh Incompatibility?

1. The medical histories of intrauterine fetal distress or neonatal jaundice, along with an indirect Coomb's test result which is positive at a ratio greater than 1:64 until the 20th week of gestation, and exceeding 1:128 for gestation weeks 20 and beyond in instances of Rh blood group incompatibilities, will necessitate a Plasma exchange
2. Plasma exchange with 5% albumin supplementation or double filtration plasmapheresis is selected, as the objective of the treatment is not to supplement coagulation factors but to eliminate antibodies
3. Till the availability of intrauterine fetal blood transfusions, the antibody titre should be kept at 1:512 or less
4. All of the above

Q14. Which of the following is true in case of Dilated cardiomyopathy (DCM)?

1. Autoimmune disorders are one of the causes of dilated cardiomyopathy (DCM)
2. Immunoglobulin G3 subclass antibodies might have a role in the pathogenesis of DCM while IgG3 is the main target of apheresis
3. Immunoadsorption plasmapheresis (IAPP) is a therapeutic apheresis treatment for DCM
4. All of the above

Q15. Which of the following is false in case of Dilated cardiomyopathy?

1. In 1996, Wallukat et al. first reported that the level of b 1 adrenergic receptor antibodies in the serum of patients with DCM was decreased by IAPP
2. In patients with DCM, a high titre of IgG3 subclass antibody is related to decreased left ventricular function
3. Imsorba TR ® is preferred for IAPP compared to Goat IgG antibody (Therasorb ®), or protein A (Immunosorba ®) as the latter requires immunoglobulin supplementation and the affinity of ligands for IgG3 is weak
4. None of the above

Q16. Which among the following is NOT associated with an increase risk of acute antibody mediated rejection in a heart transplant?

1. Young age
2. Sensitisation to muromonab (CD3)
3. History of congenital heart disease
4. Prior infection with Ebstein Bar Virus

Q17. Which among the following is the most common type of graft rejection in heart transplants?

1. Hyperacute rejection
2. Acute antibody mediated rejection
3. Acute cellular rejection
4. Chronic rejection

Q18. Which among the following statements is false with respect to therapeutic apheresis in heart transplant?

1. Extra corporeal Photopheresis (ECP) reduces production of effector T-cells while expanding Tregs (CD4+/ CD25+/Foxp3+) which suppress the immune system
2. Monotherapy with TPE is recommended for desensitisation
3. The recommended frequency of ECP is once weekly and of TPE is daily/ every other day
4. None of the above

Q19. Which among the following has been added as a new fact sheet in ASFA 2023 guidelines?

1. Intestine Transplantion
2. Autoimmune fasciitis
3. Transplantation of composite tissue
4. Pancreatic transplantation

Q20. You are conducting the initial plasmapheresis procedure on a 57-year-old male patient who is suspected of experiencing humoral rejection of a heart transplant. The procedure involves the use of albumin replacement with a goal of exchanging 1.5 plasma volumes. As the procedure nears its conclusion, the patient starts to express discomfort in the form of chest pain, prompting you to conclude the procedure prematurely after only 1.2 plasma volumes have been exchanged. After a thorough evaluation, the patient's physician determines that the chest pain is unrelated to the procedure and requests that you carry out another procedure the following day. In the interim, she asks you to calculate the fraction of the patient's intravascular antibodies that were removed. Assuming an ideal exchange, what fraction of the patient's plasma volume have you effectively replaced?

1. 22%
2. 27%
3. 37%
4. 73%

Q21. As per the American Society for Apheresis (ASFA) which of the following conditions falls into the Category IV indication, not showing any proven benefit of therapeutic plasma exchange (TPE)?

1. Stiff-person syndrome (SPS)
2. Polyneuropathy with IgG/IgA monoclonal protein
3. Chronic Inflammatory Demyelinating Polyneuropathy (CIDP)
4. Sickle cell disease (Acute stroke)

Q22. The efficacy of apheresis was observed for the following rare diseases except

1. Isaac's syndrome, Refsum's disease
2. Paraneoplastic cerebellar degeneration, HTLV-1-associated myelopathy
3. Acute disseminated encephalomyelitis, Rasmussen's encephalitis
4. None of the above

Q23. Which of the following is false regarding aging?

1. The Roman playwright Terentius claimed, "senectus ipsa est morbus" (old age itself is a disease)
2. Cicero, wrote *De Senectute*, argued, "pugnandum, tamquam contra morbum sic contra senectutem" (we must fight against aging as we do against a disease)
3. Heterochronic parabiosis model is now proposed in humans
4. None of the above

Q24. Which of the following is true with respect to aging?

1. H*eterochronic parabiosis* (blood sharing between young and old individuals leads to multitissue rejuvenation) is achieved by means of Therapeutic Plasma exchange
2. *TPE* has emerged as a potential medical intervention capable of affecting multiple pathophysiologies
3. Sham-controlled clinical trials are needed to establish TPE as treatment and/or prevention for aging and one completed trial has been reported
4. All of the above

Q25. Treating the pathophysiology in aging, which includes treatment with TPE is useful for correcting:

1. Chronic inflammation
2. Cellular senescence
3. Immunosenescence
4. *Inflammaging*(includes Chronic inflammation Cellular senescence Immunosenescence)

Q26. Which of the following is true in Alzheimer's disease?

1. A large, controlled clinical trial of TPE in Alzheimer's disease was recently published
2. It demonstrated that TPE was able to arrest the progression of the disease in patients with *moderate to severe disease* in over 60% of treated patients
3. Patients with *mild* Alzheimer's disease exhibited no progression (100%) and experienced improvements in neurophysiological aspects and also quality of life, indicating TPE has the potential to delay the development of the disease
4. All of the above

Q27. CRRT can work on which of the following?

1. Continous venovenous hemofiltration-Convection
2. Continous venovenous hemodialysis- Diffusion
3. Continous venovenous hemodiafiltration-Diffusion and Convection
4. Either of the above

Q28. CRRT in the Fig-IX-2 **is based on Continous Hemodialysis, Continous Hemofiltration, Continous Hemodiafiltration;the other modes include:**

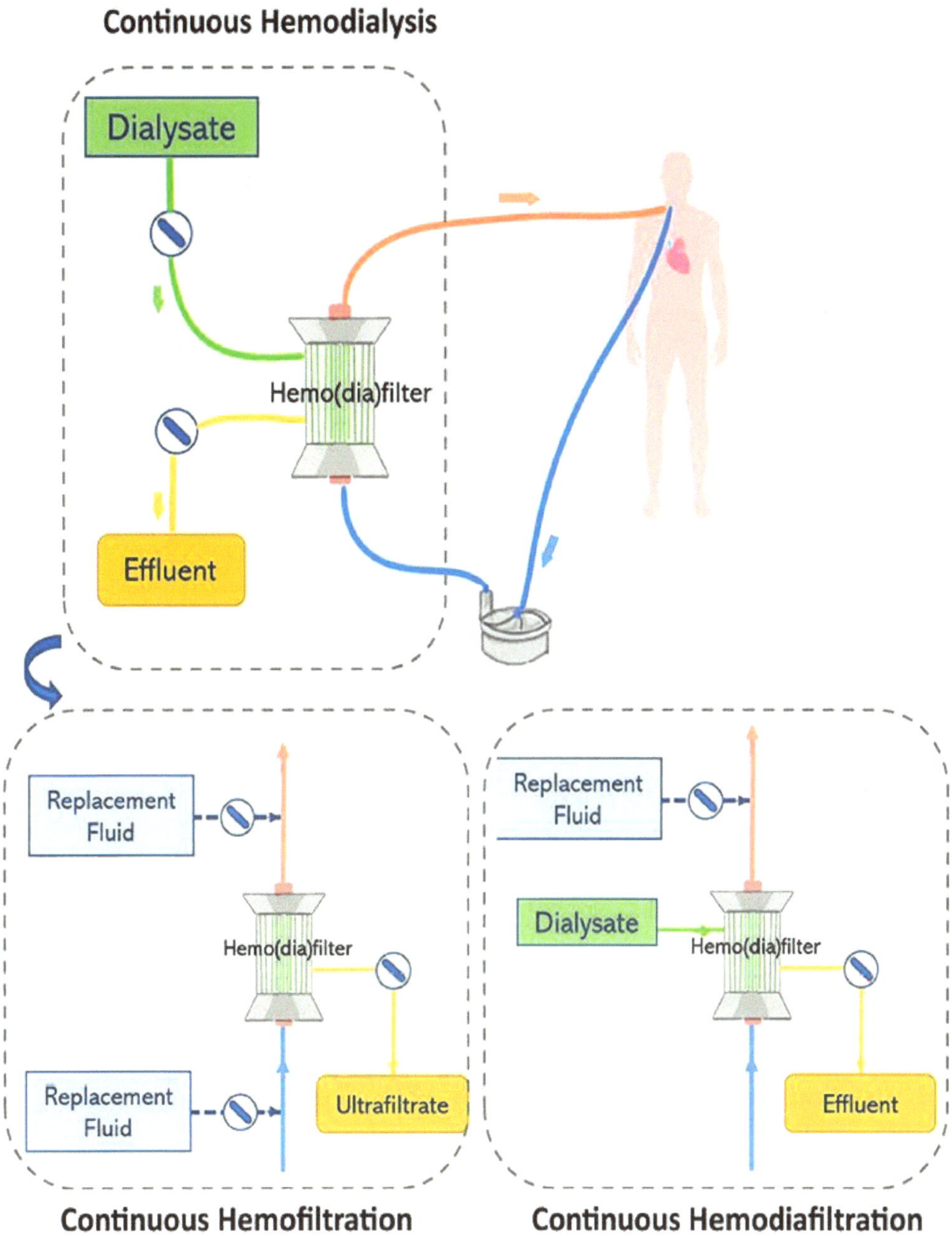

Fig-IX-2: The renal replacement therapy circuit while providing continuous hemodialysis, continuous hemofiltration, and continuous hemodiafiltration. Replacement fluid can be delivered before or after the hemofilter. reproduced from (Martins Costa, et al (12) 2022, CCBY4.0)

1. Continous Veno-Venous Hemofiltration (CVVH)- Sterile Replacement fluid is used
2. Continuous veno-hemodiafiltration(CVHDF)- Dialysate and replacement fluid is used
3. Slow continuous ultrafiltration (SCUF)- No dialysate or replacement fluid is used
4. All of the above

Q29. In case of continuous renal replacement therapy (CRRT), which of the following is true?

1. Right internal jugular vein-Most preferred site of catheter placement with Least incidence of catheter malfunction
2. Left internal jugular vein- Least preferred side of catheter placement with Highest incidence of catheter malfunction
3. Subclavian vein placement is not recommended because of likelihood to cause central venous stenosis
4. All of the above

Q30. The following is the criteria for diagnosis of AKI (acute kidney injury) except:
1. KDIGO- Increase in Serum Creatinine SCr ≥ 26.5 μmol/L within 48 h or ≥ 50% within 7d
2. RIFLE- Increase in Serum Creatinine (SCr) ≥ 50% within 7 days
3. AKIN-Increase in Serum Creatinine SCr ≥ 26.5 μmol/L or ≥ 50% within 48 hours
4. None of the above

Q31. Continuous Renal Replacement Therapy (CRRT) is a slow and continuous extracorporeal blood purification therapy. The indications include which of the following?
1. Volume overload
2. Metabolic acidosis
3. Acute Kidney injury
4. All of the above

Q32. Which of the following are recommended blood flow (Qb) rates for CRRT based on body weight?
1. 0–10 Kg; 20–60ml/min
2. 11–20 Kg; 50–100 ml/min
3. >50 Kg; 150–250 ml/min
4. All of the above

ANSWERS

Q1. Ans(4)

Q2. Ans(2)

Q3. Ans(4)

Q4. Ans(3)

Q5. Ans(3)
TPE is category III indication with 2B recommendation.

Q6. Ans(4)

Q7. Ans(4)

Q8. Ans(2)
The research examined if incorporating plasma exchange was more beneficial than administering intravenous methylprednisolone for achieving renal recovery in patients with ANCA vasculitis who had a serum creatinine level of 500 micro mol/L (5.8 mg/dl). The findings indicated a greater rate of renal recovery and independence from dialysis following plasma exchange compared to the addition of intravenous methylprednisolone in patients suffering from ANCA vasculitis.

Q9. Ans(4)

Q10. Ans(4)

Q11. Ans(4)

Q12. Ans(4)

Q13. Ans(4)

Q14. Ans(4)

Q15. Ans(4)

Q16. Ans(4)
Prior cytomegalovirus exposure increases the risk of AMR in heart transplant.

Q17. Ans(3)

Q18. Ans(2)
Neither ECP nor TPE is recommended as a monotherapy in desensitization, rejection prophylaxis, or AMR.

Q19. Ans(1)
The following conditions were incorporated into new fact sheets in ASFA 2023 updated guidelines.
- Alzheimer's disease
- Autoimmune dysautonomia
- Idiopathic inflammatory myopathies
- Immune checkpoint inhibitors, immune-related adverse events
- Paraneoplastic autoimmune retinopathies
- Transplantation, intestine
- Vaccine-induced immune thrombotic thrombocytopenia

Q20. Ans(4)

Q21. Ans(1)

Q22. Ans(4)

Q23. Ans(4)

Q24. Ans(4)

Q25. Ans(4)

Q26. Ans(4)

Q27. Ans(4)

Q28. Ans(4)

Q29. Ans(4)

Q30. Ans(4)

Q31. Ans(4)

Q32. Ans(4)

REFERENCES

1. Noiri E. and Hanafusa N., The Concise Manual of Apheresis Therapy. Tokyo:Springer Japan;2014
2. Connelly-Smith L, Alquist CR, Aqui NA, Hofmann JC, Klingel R, Onwuemene OA, Patriquin CJ, Pham HP, Sanchez AP, Schneiderman J, Witt V, Zantek ND, Dunbar NM. Guidelines on the Use of Therapeutic Apheresis in Clinical Practice - Evidence-Based Approach from the Writing Committee of the American Society for Apheresis: The Ninth Special Issue. J Clin Apher. 2023 Apr;38(2):77-278. doi: 10.1002/jca.22043. PMID: 37017433.
3. Jayne DR, Gaskin G, Rasmussen N, Abramowicz D, Ferrario F, Guillevin L, Mirapeix E, Savage CO, Sinico RA, Stegeman CA, Westman KW, van der Woude FJ, de Lind van Wijngaarden RA, Pusey CD; European Vasculitis Study Group. Randomized trial of plasma exchange or high-dosage methylprednisolone as adjunctive therapy for severe renal vasculitis. J Am Soc Nephrol. 2007;18(7):2180-8.
4. Hanafusa N et al Successful treatment by double filtrate plasmapheresis in a pregnant woman with the rare P blood group and a history of multiple early miscarriages. Ther Apher Dial 2006;10(6):498–503
5. McLeod BC, Szczepiorkowski ZM, Weinstein R, Winters JL, editors. Apheresis: Principles and Practice. 3rd ed. Bethesda, MD: AABB; 2010.
6. Kozanoglu. I., *Problem Solving in Apheresis Medicine*, Switzerland:Springer Nature; 2024.
7. Kiprov DD. Intermittent heterochronic plasma exchange as a modality for delaying cellular senescence—a hypothesis. J Clin Apher. 2013;28:387–9..
8. Boada M, Lopez OL, Olazaran J, et al. Neuropsychological, neuropsychiatric, and quality-of-life assessments in Alzheimer's disease patients treated with plasma exchange with albumin replacement from the randomized AMBAR study. Alzheimers Dement. 2022;18(7):1314–2324.
9. Singh A.K. *Core Concepts in Dialysis and Continuous Therapies.* Switzerland:Springer.:2016.
10. *RIFLE* Renal Injury Failure Loss ESRD, *AKIN* Acute Kidney Injury Network, *KDIGO* Kidney Disease Global Outcomes
11. Li Z, et al. Identification and predicting short-term prognosisof early cardiorenal syndrome type 1: KDIGO is superior to RIFLE or AKIN. PLoS One. 2014;9(12):e114369.
12. Martins Costa, A., Halfwerk, F., Wiegmann, B., Neidlin, M., & Arens, J. (2022). Trends, Advantages and Disadvantages in Combined Extracorporeal Lung and Kidney Support From a Technical Point of View. *Frontiers in Medical Technology*, *4*, 909990.p.7.
13. Cervantes, C.E.; Bloch, E.M.; Sperati, C.J. Therapeutic Plasma Exchange: Core Curriculum 2023. Am. J. Kidney Dis. 2023, 81, 475–492.
14. Mehdipour, M.; Etienne, J.; Liu, C.; Mehdipour, T.; Kato, C.; Conboy, M.; Conboy, I.; Kiprov, D.D. Attenuation of Age-Elevated Blood Factors by Repositioning Plasmapheresis: A Novel Perspective and Approach. Transfus. Apher. Sci. 2021, 60, 103162.

Chapter 11

HAEMATOPOIETIC STEM CELL TRANSPLANT (HSCT)

Dr. Swapna, Dr. Haripriya and Dr. Priyanka

Q1. Which one of the following is false in the history of transplants?

1. Indian surgeon Sushruta, performed the first plastic surgery operations
2. By the 1950s, skin grafts were the only successful transplants performed
3. The first significant governmental involvement in transplant was the National Uniform Anatomical Gift Act, was drafted in 1957
4. In 1967, Dr. Christian Barnard performed the first human to human heart transplant

Q2. Which of the following regarding the mobilization of HPC(A) Collections for Autologous Hematopoietic Cell Transplant is true?

1. Administration of G-CSF (filgrastim and lenograstim) is the available treatment option for steady-state mobilization
2. GM-CSF is no longer available in many countries
3. The other growth factors (e.g., pegylated G-CSF) have no label for PB CD34+ cell mobilization
4. All of the above

Q3. The mechanism of action of G-CSF includes which of the following?

1. Granulocyte activation and expansion and release of various proteases into the marrow
2. The proteases cleave adhesion molecules such as stromal-derived factor-1 (SDF-1), releasing hematopoietic stem and progenitor cells (specifically CD34+ cells) into the peripheral Blood
3. In normal circumstances, CD34+ cells circulate in very small numbers in the peripheral blood
4. All of the above

Q4. Which of the following is true for mobilization in case of Autologous HSCT?

1. Filgrastim and lenograstim are usually injected at a daily dose of 10 μg/kg of body weight subcutaneously
2. The approved schedules of G-CSF are 5–7 consecutive days for filgrastim and 4–6 days for lenograstim
3. Leukapheresis should be started at least on days 5 or 6 after filgrastim and between days 5 and 7 after lenograstim
4. All of the above

Q5. Which of the following statements regarding adverse events associated with granulocyte colony-stimulating factor (G-CSF) administration is false?

1. Serious adverse events, such as splenic rupture, have been reported following G-CSF administration in healthy donors and patients
2. G-CSF administration is associated with an average increase of approximately 11 mm in splenic length and a 10% increase in splenic volume
3. Splenic rupture occurs in the majority of subjects on day 6 of G-CSF administration
4. None of the above

Q6. The adverse effects of G- CSF include which of the following?

1. A procoagulant effect
2. A probable increased risk of myocardial infarction
3. A probable increased risk of ischaemic strokes in susceptible individuals
4. All of the above

Q7. Which of the following are recombinant human G-CSF?

1. Peg-GCSF
2. Filgrastim
3. Lenograstim
4. All of the above

Q8. Which of the following is true regarding G-CSF administration?

1. The twice daily subcutaneous injection is more efficient in mobilizing PBSC in normal donors than is a single injection
2. The twice daily subcutaneous injection requires fewer apheresis procedures without increasing toxicity
3. The G-CSF injection is continued if the target CD34+ cell yield is not achieved
4. All of the above

Q9. Which of the following are true regarding mobilisation with Plerixafor except

1. Plerixafor is a reversible chemokine receptor 4 (CXCR4) antagonist when used in combination with G-CSF increases the CD34+ cells release from the bone marrow by interrupting with the binding of CXCR4 and stromal cell-derived factor-1 (SDF-1)
2. The recommended dose is 240 μg/kg body weight subcutaneously
3. It is administered about 24 h before initiation of leukapheresis following at least 4 days of G-CSF pretreatment
4. In patients with impaired renal function (creatinine clearance ≤ 50 mL/min), dose adjustment to 160 μg/kg b.w. is recommended

Q10. Plerixafor can be used in combination with G- CSF in patients who have previously failed mobilisation, What is the success rate?

1. 50%
2. 60%
3. 70%
4. 80%

Q11. Which of the following is true with respect to Hematopoietic progenitor cells(HPC)?

1. The circulating HPCs comprise about 0.1% of the total white blood cell count in the steadystate
2. CD34 is a highly glycosylated phosphor glycoprotein expressed on progenitor cells of all lineages within the lympho-haemopoietic system and is a surrogate marker for stem cells
3. Approximately 0.5% of cord blood cells are CD34+
4. All of the above

Q12. Which among the following is false regarding mobilisation?

1. The number of CD34+ cells infused clearly correlates with both neutrophil and platelet recovery post-transplant
2. G-CSF mobilised grafts contain 3–4-fold higher CD34+ cells compared to marrow harvests
3. G-CSF mobilised grafts contain 10–20-fold increase in CD3+ T cells compared with marrow harvests
4. None of the above

Q13. Which of the following is true regarding G-CSF administration?

1. After G-CSF administration, both the complete blood count (CBC) and the white blood cell (WBC) fraction are examined
2. If WBC exceeds 50,000 cells/ μ L, the G-CSF dose is reduced
3. If WBC exceeds 75,000 cells/ μ L, the G-CSF injections are stopped
4. All of the above

Q14. In PBSC Collection, which of the following are true?

1. When CD 34+ counts not available, increase of monocyte rates, reticulocyte numbers, and LDH values are used as predictive factors for the CD34+ cell yield
2. When there is a sharp increase in WBC compared with that of the previous day (for example, 500 to 2,500/ μ L), there is a possibility of achieving sufficient CD34+ cells even if the total WBC is lower than 2,500/ μ L
3. Hematopoietic progenitor cell (HPC) quantifications are also used to predict the timing of CD34+ cell mobilization
4. All of the above

Q15. Peripheral Blood Haematopoietic Progenitor Cell Collection (Leucocytapheresis) following chemotherapy and G- CSF mobilisation, can commence if

1. Leucocyte counts are rising ($\geq 1 \times 10^9$/L)
2. Leucocyte counts are rising ($\geq 5 \times 10^9$/L)
3. Leucocyte counts are rising ($\geq 15 \times 10^9$/L)
4. Leucocyte counts are rising ($\geq 20 \times 10^9$/L)

Q16. Which of the following is false regarding collection of Hematopoietic cells?

1. Lansky was able to collect sufficient number of pluripotent hematopoietic cells from normal donors by apheresis in 1982
2. Kessinger showed the ability of peripheral blood-derived hematopoietic progenitor cells to restore normal haematopoiesis after chemotherapy-associated aplasia in breast cancer patients
3. Barlogie et al. used autologous bone marrow derived HSCT in refractory multiple myeloma
4. None of the above

Q17. The targets for collections in HSCT include which of the following?

1. For the autologous setting anywhere in the ranges of $2–5 \times 10^6$ CD34+ cells/kg
2. For allogeneic transplants is usually in the range of $4–8 \times 10^6$ CD34+ cells/kg of recipient weight.
3. These doses are achieved by processing a fixed volume of blood per collection (e.g., 2–3 blood volumes)
4. All of the above

Q18. Which among the following is false in PBSC collection?

1. Blood prime is needed for individuals with small stature or anemia as they are more vulnerable to changes in hematocrit during a procedure
2. Since only a few milliliters of the priming unit enter the patient ́s circulation, blood priming has little effect on the collection yield (dilutional effect)
3. Optimizing hematocrit prior to collection and priming the apheresis circuit with RBCs diminishes the changes in extra corporeal volume and post-procedure hematocrit, resulting in fewer adverse events
4. None of the above

Q19. Which of the following is best to consider for Stem cells collection (rather than just CD34+ cell or MNC yield)?

1. A product with a high percentage of MNC and a low percentage of granulocytes suggests that the collection was appropriate
2. High granulocyte and RBC counts suggest that the collection was too deep and the buffy coat containing the target cells was not harvested
3. A high platelet content and low overall WBC and RBC contents would indicate that the collection was too large, and the required cells were missing from the buffy coat
4. All of the above

Q20. The required number of CD34+ cells for allogeneic transplants is increased

1. If there is increased human leucocyte antigen (HLA) disparity between donor and recipient
2. In case of Tandem transplant
3. In case of Graft manipulation
4. All of the above

Q21. Large- volume leucocytapheresis (processing of 3–6 blood volumes over a longer period of time or by increasing the blood flow into the apheresis machine) may collect more CD34+ cells. Which of the following is true?

1. Donor inconvenience, citrate toxicity and platelet loss are some of the side effects
2. It is successfully used for allogeneic donors
3. It is used successfully for poorly mobilising autologous patients
4. All of the above

Q22. For the collection of Stem cells, which of the following is true?

1. The Spectra Optia was approved by the FDA for harvesting HPC(A) in 2012 using the Mono Nuclear Cells protocol and 2015 using the Continuous Mono Nuclear Cells protocol
2. The MNC content indicates if the collection was drawn from the appropriate layer
3. Etiology of unexpected hematopoietic graft yields and product content can happen due to patient/donor characteristics, operator errors, and equipment malfunction
4. All of the above

Q23. Passenger Lymphocyte Syndrome presents with delayed hemolysis in which of the following incompatible Hematopoietic stem progenitor cells transplant (HCT)?

1. Major ABO I HCT
2. Minor ABO I HCT
3. Bidirectional HCT
4. 2&3

Q24. For Passenger Lymphocyte Syndrome in case of Minor ABO Mismatch, which of the following is true?

1. It is a serious complication which may occur between days +5 and +15 of transplant
2. The high iso- hemagglutinin titres cause acute anemia and therapeutic plasma exchange (TPE) is required to reduce the high titres
3. Delayed hemolysis (up to 4 months) of residual recipient RBCs by donor-derived iso hemagglutinins occurs and it is mainly self-limiting and resolves spontaneously
4. All of the above

Q25. Which of the following are true for allo HCT for Beta Thalassemia Major (BTM)?

1. The cure of BTM by bone marrow transplantation was first demonstrated by Thomas et al.
2. Transplant-related risk factors should be evaluated according to the Pesaro risk score
3. Pretransplant preparation of these patients includes myeloablative and immunosuppressive treatment in order to overcome the barriers to a successful allo-HCT
4. All of the above

Q26. Regarding the treatment for Thalassemia, which of the following is true?

1. Theoretically, all patients affected with Transfusion Dependant Thalassemia (TDT) are candidates for allo-HCT
2. Allo-HCT is offered as soon as possible in patients with transfusion dependent thalassemia
3. Matched sibling donors and Matched sibling umbilical cord are the allogeneic sources
4. All of the above

Q27. Indications for Allo-HCT in Sickle cell Anemia include which of the following?

1. Stroke
2. Recurrent severe acute chest syndrome (ACS) –especially with episodes of respiratory failure
3. Chronic ongoing or acute intermittent debilitating vaso-occlusive episode interfering with lifestyle
4. All of the above

Q28. Which of the following is false in the management of Aplastic Anemia?

1. For newly diagnosed cases of aplastic anemia (AA) patients, upfront treatment option includes either allogeneic hematopoietic stem cell transplant (HSCT) or immunosuppressive therapy (IST)
2. Currently, the decision to select HSCT or IST as upfront treatment is based on patients age and availability of a human leukocyte antigen (HLA) matched donor
3. Preferred donor source in order of priority is - Matched related donor (preferably ABO compatible), Matched unrelated donor and Related haploidentical donor
4. None of the above

Q29. The incidence of culture-positive HPC (A) products reported in the literature ranges from

1. 0 to 7.2%, but is typically <1–2%
2. 0 to 8.5%, but is typically <3%
3. 0 to 6%, but is typically <4%
4. 0 to 5% , but is typically <1–2%

Q30. Hematocrit of the HPC (A) product is usually in the range of______?

1. 2–4%
2. 10-15%
3. 15- 20%
4. 25-30%

Q31. In cases of major ABO-mismatched Hematopoietic Progenitor Cell (HPC) transplantation, if incompatible red cells cannot be removed from the HPCproduct, Therapeutic Plasma Exchange (TPE) is performed to lower the relevant isoagglutinin titer to what maximum level?

1. $\leq$ 1:4
2. $\leq$ 1:8
3. $\leq$ 1:16
4. $\leq$ 1:32

Q32. Which of the following is the primary risk of failing to desensitise a patient with strongly positive DSA prior to HSCT?

1. Vaso occlusive disease
2. Graft failure
3. Delayed neutrophil recovery
4. CMV reactivation

Q33. A patient undergoing unrelated donor HSCT has moderate DSA (MFI 4,000). The transplant team plans desensitisation with TPE. According to ASFA 2023 guidelines, what is the ASFA category for TPE in HLA desensitisation prior to HSCT?

1. Category I
2. Category II
3. Category III
4. Category IV

Q34. A 56-year-old man awaiting allogeneic HSCT for MDS has DSA of MFI 18,000. Despite 4sessions of TPE and rituximab, the MFI remains unchanged. What is the next step in management of this patient?

1. Increase frequency of TPE to twice daily
2. Add bortezomib to the desensitisation regimen
3. Switch to leukocytapheresis
4. Stop desensitisation and proceed to transplant

Q35. What is the MFI beyond which DSA is considered positive?

1. 100
2. 1000
3. 500
4. 10

Q36. When a donors CD34+ count reaches 30×10^6/L, a CD34 collection is initiated. The total blood volume (without anticoagulant) processed amounts to 15 L. This procedure successfully collected 4×10^6/kg based on the patients body weight of 70 kg. Please calculate the collection efficiency (CE)

1. The CE for this CD34 collection is $280/(30 \times 15) \times 100 = 62.2\%$
2. The CE for this CD34 collection is $4/(30) \times 100 = 13.3\%$
3. The CE for this CD34 collection is $4/(15) \times 100 = 26.6\%$
4. None of the above

ANSWERS

Q1. Ans(3)
The first significant governmental involvement in transplant was the National Uniform Anatomical Gift Act, was drafted in 1967.

Q2. Ans(4)

Q3. Ans(4)

Q4. Ans(4)

Q5. Ans(4)

Q6. Ans(4)

Q7. Ans(4)

Q8. Ans(4)

Q9. Ans(3)
It is administered approximately 6-11 hours before initiation of leukapheresis following at least 4 days of G-CSF pretreatment

Q10. Ans(3)

Q11. Ans(4)

Q12. Ans(4)

Q13. Ans(4)

Q14. Ans(4)

Q15. Ans(1)

Q16. Ans(4)

Q17. Ans(4)

Q18. Ans(4)

Q19. Ans(4)

Q20. Ans(4)

Q21. Ans(4)

Q22. Ans(4)

Q23. Ans(4)

Q24. Ans(4)

Q25. Ans(4)

Q26. Ans(4)

Q27. Ans(4)

Q28. Ans(4)

Q29. Ans(1)

Q30. Ans(1)

Q31. Ans(3)

Q32. Ans(2)
Explanation: High-titer DSA is strongly associated with primary graft failure.

Q33. Ans(3)

Q34. Ans(2)
Explanation: In cases with high MFI, multimodal approach helps in avoiding rebound DSA production after TPE; namely IVIG, immunoadsorption, rituximab, donor platelet/buffy coat infusions and eculizumab

Q35. Ans(2)

Q36. Ans(1)
CE2 = Cells product/[PrePBcount × (TBVprocessed-ACvolume)]* × 100
**the TBV processed – AC volume in liters*
The CE2 formula is used, since the post PB CD34+ count is unknown. It is necessary to calculate the absolute number of CD34+ cells in the collection bag. The collected value is 4×10^6/kg, the absolute number of CD34+ cells in the collection bag is 4×10^6/kg × 70 kg or 280×10^6.

REFERENCES

1. Qureshi UA, Gosain AK. Sushruta: The Father of Indian Surgical History. Plast Reconstr Surg Glob Open. 2024; 12(11):e6309.
2. Nordham KD, Ninokawa S. The history of organ transplantation. Proc (Bayl Univ Med Cent). 2021;35(1):124-128.
3. Abutalib SA, Padmanabhan A, Pham HP, Worel N, editors. Best practices of apheresis in hematopoietic cell transplantation. 2020th ed. Cham, Switzerland: Springer International Publishing; 2019
4. Giralt S, Costa L, Schriber J, DiPersio J, Maziarz R, McCarty J et al Optimizing autologous stem cell mobilization strategies to improve patient outcomes: consensus guidelines and recommendations. Biol Blood Marrow Tr 2014;20(3):295–308.
5. Pusic I, DiPersio JF The use of growth factors in hematopoietic stem cell transplantation. Curr Pharm Des 2008;14(20):1950–1961
6. Murphy MF, Roberts DJ, Mark H, Yazer NM, editors. Practical Transfusion Medicine Sixth Edition. Hoboken, NJ: John Wiley & Sons, Inc; 2022.
7. Kröger N, Renges H, Krüger W et al A randomized comparison of once versus twice daily recombinant human granulocyte colony-stimulating factor (filgrastim) for stem cell mobilization in healthy donors for allogeneic transplantation. BrJ Haematol 2000;111:761–765

8. Lee V, Li CK, Shing MM et al Single vs twice daily G-CSFdose for peripheral blood stem cells harvest in normal donors andchildren with non-malignant diseases. Bone Marrow Transplant 2000;25:931–935
9. Noiri E.and Hanafusa N., The Concise Manual of Apheresis Therapy. Tokyo: Springer Japan;2014
10. Pahnke S, Egeland T, Halter J et al. Current use of biosimilar G- CSF for haematopoietic stem cell mobilization. Bone Marrow Transplant 2019;54:858–66.
11. NHS England. Clinical commissioning policy: use of plerixafor for stem cell mobilization (update). https:// www. england.nhs.uk/publication/ plerixafor- for-stem- cell- mobilisation- in- adults- and- children
12. Kawakami K, Abe Y, Imataki O et al. Determining the time of harvesting peripheral blood stem cells using the HPC, for monitoring hematopoietic progenitor cells, of the automated hematology analyzer XE-2100. Sysmex J 2006;29:39–45
13. Lasky LC, Ash RC, Kersey JH, et al. Collection of pluripotential hematopoietic stem cells by cytapheresis. Blood. 1982;59:822–7.
14. Kessinger A, Armitage JO, Landmark JD, et al. Reconstitution of human hematopoietic function with autologous cryopreserved circulating stem cells. Exp Hematol. 1986;14:192–6.
15. Barlogie B, Alexanian R, Dicke KA, et al. High-dose chemoradiotherapy and autologous bone marrow transplantation for resistant multiple myeloma. Blood. 1987;70:869–72.
16. Cherqaoui B, Rouel N, Auvrignon A, Defachelles AS, Demeocq F, Kanold J, et al. Peripheral blood stem cell collection in low-weight children: retrospective comparison of two apheresis devices. Transfusion. 2014;54(5):1371–8.
17. Ohara Y, Ohto H, Tasaki T, Sano H, Mochizuki K, Akaihata M, et al. Comprehensive technical and patient-care optimization in the management of pediatric apheresis for peripheral blood stem cell harvesting. Transfus Apher Sci. 2016;55(3):338–43.
18. Kozanoglu I., *Problem Solving in Apheresis Medicine*, Switzerland:Springer Nature; 2024.
19. Mohty M, Hubel K, Kroger N et al. Autologous haematopoietic stem cell mobilization in multiple myeloma and lymphoma patients; a position statement from the European Group for Blood and Marrow Transplantation. Bone Marrow Transplant 2014;49:865–72.
20. Hubel K. Mobilization and collection of HSC. In E Carreras, C Dufour, M Mohty, N Kroger (eds), The EBMT Handbook. Cham: Springer Open, 2019: 117–22. https://www.ebmt.org/education/ ebmt- handbook
21. Thomas ED, Buckner CD, Sanders JE, Papayannopoulou T, Borgna-Pignatti C, De Stefano P, et al. Marrow transplantation for thalassaemia. Lancet 1982;2:227-9.
22. R Iftikhar, QUN Chaudhry, F Anwer. Allogeneic hematopoietic stem cell transplantation in aplastic anemia: current indications and transplant strategies. Blood Rev, 2021;47 , p. 100772
23. Abutalib SA. Clinical manual of blood and bone marrow transplantation [Internet]. Abutalib SA, Hari P, editors. Nashville, TN: John Wiley & Sons; 2017.
24. McLeod BC, Szczepiorkowski ZM, Weinstein R, Winters JL, editors. Apheresis: Principles and Practice. 3rd ed. Bethesda, MD: AABB; 2010.
25. Connelly-Smith L, Alquist CR, Aqui NA, Hofmann JC, Klingel R, Onwuemene OA, Patriquin CJ, Pham HP, Sanchez AP, Schneiderman J, Witt V, Zantek ND, Dunbar NM. Guidelines on the Use of Therapeutic Apheresis in Clinical Practice - Evidence-Based Approach from the Writing Committee of the American Society for Apheresis: The Ninth Special Issue. J Clin Apher. 2023 Apr;38(2):77-278. doi: 10.1002/jca.22043. PMID: 37017433.
26. Ciurea, S.O., Cao, K., Fernandez-Vina, M. *et al.* The European Society for Blood and Marrow Transplantation (EBMT) Consensus Guidelines for the Detection and Treatment of Donor-specific Anti-HLA Antibodies (DSA) in Haploidentical Hematopoietic Cell Transplantation. *Bone Marrow Transplant* 53,2018; 521–534

Chapter 12

EXTRACORPOREAL PHOTOPHERESIS

Dr. Swapna and Dr. Priyanka

Q1. Which among the following is false in the history of Extracorporeal Photopheresis ECP?

1. In ancient Egypt, patients with vitiligo ingested a plant (Ammi majus) from the banks of the Nile, bathed in the sun and noticed recovery in melanin production
2. Edelson et al. was one of the first scientists to develop ECP as a treatment for patients with cutaneous T-cell lymphoma (CTCL)
3. 1988, the US Food and Drug Administration approved ECP
4. None of the above

Q2. Which of the following is false in the process of ECP?

1. This procedure combines leukocytapheresis, treatment of cells with ultraviolet A (UVA) light after exposure to 8-methoxypsoralen, and reinfusion into the patient
2. This therapy is used in the treatment of autoimmune syndromes, cutaneous T-cell lymphoma, graft-versus-host disease, and cell-mediated rejection following solid-organ transplantation
3. The use of psoralen and UVA light crosslinks nucleic acids, causing disruption of DNA transcription and replication
4. None of the above

Q3. Mechanism of action of Extracorporeal Photopheresis includes which of the following?

1. This process has no known immunosuppressive effect and leads to immune tolerance by increasing the number of regulatory T cells (Tregs)
2. More than two million procedures have been performed but the mechanism of action is not understood clearly
3. Its efficacy is mainly related to the apoptosis of lymphocytes and differentiation of dendritic cells
4. All of the above

Q4. ECP is contraindicated in which of the following conditions?

1. Patients with sensitivity to psoralen products and known photosensitivity
2. Patients presenting with a risk of retinal damage, pregnancy, hemodynamic instability, respiratory instability
3. Patients with low leukocyte count ($<1 \times 10^9$/L) despite granulocyte colony-stimulating factor)
4. Patients with normal platelet count and absence of infection

Q5. Which of the following is false for a requirement of ECP?

1. There is still no recommendation of minimum number of cells to be processed per ECP session or amount of blood volume to be processed for collection of cells
2. At least 1×10^9 /L cells in the peripheral blood are required before initiating the ECP therapy
3. However, cell dosage from as low as 3.3×10^8 (mini ECP) up to 2.8×10^9 were reported with adequate clinical response in patients
4. None of the above

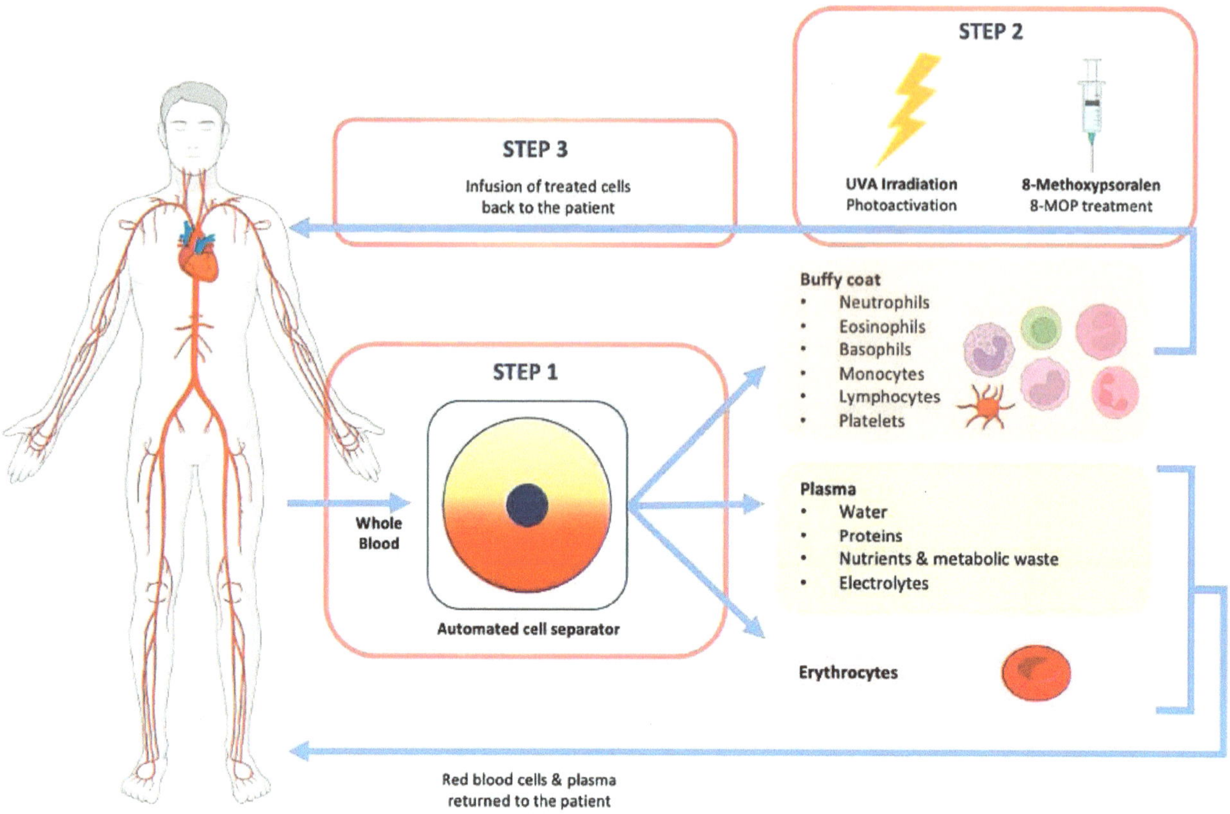

Fig-X-1: Overview of the ECP procedure,
(reproduced from Bojanic, I., Worel, N., Pacini, C. P., Stary, G., et al (15) 2023, CCBY4.0)

Q6. Which of the following instruments is used for ECP mechanism indicated in Fig X-1:
1. CELLEX™
2. UVAR-XTS™
3. The Amicus™ Separator (Fresenius Kabi, Germany)
4. All of the above

Q7. Which of the following is false in the validation of ECP?
1. Validation of 8-MOP
2. Validation tests are recommended for the first two sessions of ECP in the first cycle, change of UVA illuminator, or cell separator
3. Validation of irradiation is assessed by evaluating the change in the number of 7-aminoactinomycin positive CD3+ cells within 72–96 h post-ECP
4. None of the above

Q8. Which of the following is false in ECP treatment and post procedure treatment?
1. Each session of ECP is an invasive procedure (depending on the type of method used)
2. Patient variables that should be assessed for the initiation of therapy include hemoglobin level (>10 g/dl), platelets count ($>20 \times 10^9$ /L), weight (>20 kg); specifically for "In-Line"method
3. Post-each session, the patient should be prescribed high SPF sun cream (15 or above) and UVA sunglasses (for 48 h post each session), to avoid the adverse effect of 8-MOP used
4. None of the above

Q9. Which of the following is a Food and Drug Administration (FDA) approved indication for extracorporeal photopheresis (ECP)?
1. Graft-versus-host disease (GVHD)
2. Heart transplant rejection
3. Lung transplant rejection
4. Cutaneous T-cell lymphoma

Q10. **You are asked to engage in a discussion regarding the risks associated with ECPfor a patient who intends to receive treatment for chronic graft-versus-host disease(cGVHD) following a hematopoietic progenitor cell (HPC) transplant for acute myeloidleukemia (AML). She expresses concern about the potential long-term effects of ECP, having read online that the precise mechanism through which ECP alleviates GVHDremains unclear. What is the sole known long-term side effect of repeated ECPtreatments that you inform her about?**

1. Increased risk of infection
2. Increased risk of malignancy
3. Increased risk of iron-deficiency anemia
4. Increased risk of diabetes and osteopenia

ANSWERS

Q1. Ans(4) **Q2.** Ans(4) **Q3.** Ans(4) **Q4.** Ans(4) **Q5.** Ans(4) **Q6.** Ans(4)

Q7. Ans(4) **Q8.** Ans(4) **Q9.** Ans(4) **Q10.** Ans(3)

REFERENCES

1. Heshmati F et al. Transfus Apher Sci 2003;28:25–34.
2. Edelson R, Berger C, Gasparro F, Jegasothy B, Heald P, Wintroub B, et al. Treatment ofcutaneous T-cell lymphoma by extracorporeal photochemotherapy. Preliminary results. N Engl J Med 1987;316:297-303
3. Raval JS, Ratcliffe NR. Extracorporeal photopheresis and personalized medicine in the 21st century: the future's so bright! J Clin Apher. 2018;33:461
4. Marques MB, Adamski J. Extracorporeal photopheresis: technique, established and novel indications. J Clin Apher. 2014;29(4):228–34.
5. Perfetti P, Carlier P, Strada P, et al. Extracorporeal photopheresis for the treatment of steroid-refractory acute GVHD. Bone Marrow Transplant. 2008;42:609–17.
6. Greinix HT, Volc-Platzer B, Knobler RM. Extracorporeal photochemotherapy in the treatment of severe graft-versus-host disease. Leuk Lymphoma. 2000;36(5–6):425–34.
7. Penack O, Marchetti M, Ruutu T, et al. Prophylaxis and management of graft versus host disease after stem-cell transplantation for haematological malignancies: updated consensus recommendations of the European Society for Blood and Marrow Transplantation. Lancet Haematol. 2020;7(2):e157–67.
8. Knobler R, Arenberger P, Arun A, Assaf C, Bagot M, Berlin G, et al. European dermatology forum—updated guidelines on the use of extracorporeal photopheresis 2020—part 1. J Eur Acad Dermatol Venereol. 2020;34(12):2693–716.
9. Liu C, Shah K, Dynis M, Eby CS, Grossman BJ. Linear relationship between lymphocyte counts in peripheral blood and buffy coat collected during extracorporeal photopheresis. Transfusion. 2013;53:2635–43.
10. Hackstein H, Misterek J, Nockher A, Reiter A, Bein G, Woessmann W. Mini buffy coat photopheresis for children and critically ill patients with extracorporeal photopheresis contraindications. Transfusion. 2009;49:2366–73.
11. Arora, S., & Setia, R. (2017). Extracorporeal photopheresis: Review of technical aspects. *Asian Journal of Transfusion Science*, *11*(2), 81.
12. Pierelli L, Perseghin P, Marchetti M, Messina C, Perotti C, Mazzoni A, et al. Extracorporeal photopheresis for the treatment of acute and chronic graft-versus-host disease in adults and children: Best practice recommendations from an Italian Society of Hemapheresis and Cell Manipulation (SIdEM) and Italian Group for Bone Marrow Transplantation (GITMO) consensus process. Transfusion. 2013;53:2340–52.
13. Adamski J, Ipe TS, Kinard T. Therapeutic and donor apheresis. In: Pham HP, Williams LA III, editors. *Transfusion Medicine, Apheresis, and Hemostasis: Review Questions and Case Studies*. 1st ed. London (UK): Academic Press; 2017. p. 327–352.
14. Radwanski K, Burgstaler E, Weitgenant J, Dale H, Heber C, Winters J. Pilot study of a new online extracorporeal photopheresis system in patients with steroid refractory or dependent chronic graft vs host disease. *J Clin Apheresis* (2020) 35(4):342–50.
15. Bojanic, I., Worel, N., Pacini, C. P., Stary, G., Piekarska, A., Flinn, A. M., Schell, K. J., Gennery, A. R., Knobler, R., Lacerda, J. F., Greinix, H. T., Pulanic, D., & Crossland, R. E. (2023). Extracorporeal photopheresis as an immunomodulatory treatment modality for chronic GvHD and the importance of emerging biomarkers. *Frontiers in Immunology*, *14*, 1086006. Figure 1 Overview of the ECP procedure p.2.

Chapter 13

DONOR LYMPHOCYTE INFUSION (DLI)

Dr. Shahida

Q1. Which cell type is used to calculate DLI dosing in clinical practice?
1. CD34+ cells
2. CD19+ cells
3. CD3+ cells
4. Total nucleated cells

Q2. Response following a DLI infusion is usually seen after:
1. 3 to 4 weeks
2. 3 to 4 months
3. 3 to 4 years
4. 6 months

Q3. The principle therapeutic effect of DLI is mediated by:
1. Graft versus Leukemia effect
2. Myeloablation
3. Stem cell rescue
4. Cytokine wash out

Q4. Most common major complication of DLI is:
1. Veno-occlusive disease
2. Acute graft-versus-host disease
3. Infusion associated infections
4. Tumor lysis syndrome

Q5. Which relapse setting shows the HIGHEST response rates to DLI?
1. Acute lymphoblastic leukemia
2. Acute myeloid leukemia
3. Chronic myeloid leukemia
4. Plasma cell leukemia

Q6. Pre-emptive DLI is most appropriately used for:
1. After Primary graft failure
2. After Overt haematological relapse
3. When Minimal residual disease is detected
4. When Severe chronic GVHD is developed

Q7. Which immunologic mechanism contributes to reduced GVHD after delayed DLI?
1. Loss of donor T cells
2. Development of immune tolerance
3. Reduced antigen presentation
4. Depletion of NK cells

Q8. Factors influencing GVHD after DLI include:
1. CD3+ cell dose
2. Timing post-transplant
3. Donor recipient HLA disparity
4. ABO compatibility

Choose the right answer from the given options:
1. 1,2,3 are correct
2. 1 and 3 are correct
3. 2 and 4 are correct
4. All are correct

Q9. Strategies improving safety of haplo-DLI include all EXCEPT:
1. Dose escalation
2. Short term immunosuppression
3. MRD guided administration
4. Avoiding GVHD monitoring

Q10. All of the following are TRUE regarding DLI except:
1. Is a form of cellular therapy
2. Mobilization is required for collection
3. Same donor who provided the cells for HSCT is used
4. For each collection, the donor needs to undergo eligibility testing

Q11. The most cell population responsible for the therapeutic effect of DLI is:
1. CD34+ hematopoetic stem cells
2. CD3+ T lymphocytes
3. CD19+ B lymphocytes
4. Natural Killer Cells

Q12. An ACTIVE graft versus host disease is considered as a:
1. Strong indication for DLI
2. Relative indication for DLI
3. Relative contraindication for DLI
4. Absolute contraindication for DLI

Q13. Which disease setting shows the POOREST response to DLI?
1. Molecular relapse of CML
2. Mixed donor chimerism
3. Overt relapse of acute leukemia
4. Cytogenetic relapse of CML

Q14. A key rationale for dose escalated DLI schedule is to:
1. Increase stem cell engraftment
2. Prevent marrow aplasia
3. Reduce GVHD while preserving GVL
4. Eliminate the need for immunosuppression

Q15. Which timing of DLI is associated with LOWER GVHD risk?
1. Within 30 days of post-HSCT
2. During active immunosuppression
3. Early post-transplant period
4. Delayed administration after immune reconstitution

Q16. Which clinical scenario is appropriate for Prophylactic DLI?
1. High risk disease with mixed chimerism
2. Overt relapse with high tumor burden
3. Primary graft failure
4. Presence of minimal residual disease

Q17. Compared with matched donor DLI, Haploidentical DLI:
1. Is contraindicated
2. Can be safely used with lower starting doses
3. Has universally higher GVHD rates
4. Is ineffective

Q18. Which monitoring parameter is important after DLI administration?

1. Serum ferritin
2. Chimerism status
3. Reticulocyte count
4. Serum calcium

Q19. Marrow aplasia following DLI is MOST likely when DLI is given to patients with:

1. Full donor chimerism
2. Mixed chimerism
3. Predominant host hematopoiesis
4. Prior chronic GVHD

Q20. Which premedication needs to be avoided during DLI administration?

1. Paracetamol
2. Chlorpheniramine
3. Hydrocortisone
4. Antihistamine

ANSWERS

Q1. Ans(3)
Explanation: EBMT guidelines recommend expressing DLI dose as CD3+ T cell per kilogram of recipient's body weight. This allows standardized dosing and better prediction of GVHD risk. Other cellular parameters are not used for dose calculation.

Q2. Ans(2)
Explanation: Depending on the disease indication, the beginning of a response is usually seen within 2 to 3 months after infusion; however, a full response may take more than 1 year.

Q3. Ans(1)
Explanation: Unmanipulated DLI is a form of immunotherapy, which can induce durable remissions by enhancing the graft-versus-tumor (GvT) or graft-versus-Leukemia (GVL) effect. DLI enhances GVT/GVL immune responses through donor T Lymphocytes.

Q4. Ans(2)
Explanation: GVHD is the dose-limiting and most frequent toxicity associated with DLI. Thus, different strategies like T cell depletion, immunotherapy with Abatacept are being explored to reduce the risk of GVHD while maintaining antitumor activity. Another strategy is to insert an inducible suicide gene in donor lymphocytes so that they can be selectively eliminated to treat DLI-associated GvHD.

Q5. Ans(3)
Explanation: Efficacy of DLI varies by type and burden of the disease. DLI is more effective in CML leading to complete remission in 70-80% of the patients in hematologic or cytogenetic CML relapse, whereas less than 40% of acute leukemia patients responds to DLI.

Q6. Ans(3)
Explanation: Pre-emptive DLI at minimal residual disease (MRD) stage achieves better disease control with less toxicity. It is important to monitor for MRD after allo-HCT as DLI is probably more effective when administered for MRD compared to overt hematologic relapse. Retrospective studies have shown that persistent MRD post-transplant is associated with high relapse rate and poor outcomes and the eradication of MRD improves survival. Thus, Close monitoring of MRD and donor chimerism after a successful therapeutic haplo-DLI is important to identify the patients who are at high-risk of subsequent relapses.

The term pre-emptive DLI is used in patients in haematological disease remission, but with incomplete or decreasing donor chimerism, or with detectable disease at a very low level, either as measurable residual disease or when the first signs of subclinical relapse are observed (eg, molecular or cytogenetic relapse), or detection of recurrent disease by flow cytometry.

Q7. Ans(2)
Explanation: Post-transplant immune tolerance lowers alloreactivity with delayed DLI. Presence of donor derived tolerogenic cells in the recipient may reduce their alloreactivity and thus the risk of GVHD

Q8. Ans(1)
ABO compatibility does not influence the GVHD risk. GVHD risk correlates with T cell dose and timing after HSCT. HLA disparity is relevant only in haplo-identical settings.

Q9. Ans(4)
Active GVHD monitoring is essential; all others improve safety.

Q10. Ans(2)
Explanation: Mononuclear cells (MNCs), including monocytes, lymphocytes, natural killer (NK) cells, and dendritic cells, can also be collected from the peripheral blood (MNC, Apheresis), typically from unstimulated donors, for DLI and for further processing into cellular immunotherapy products.

Q11. Ans(2)

Explanation: DLI products are enriched in donor T lymphocytes, quantified as CD3+ cells. These cells mediate both graft-versus-leukemia effects and graft versus host disease. CD34+ cells are not intentionally included in DLI.

Q12. Ans(4)

Explanation: EBMT clearly sates that Active GVHD is an absolute contraindication to DLI. Infusing donor lymphocytes in this setting significantly increases the risk of severe, life-threatening GVHD. However, a history of cortico-sensitive acute GVHD (grade 2–4), or moderate or severe chronic GVHD, are defined as relative contraindications, depending on the timing of immune suppression withdrawal, the timing of GVHD, and the risk of the underlying malignancy, and should always be discussed on a case-by-case basis.

Q13. Ans(3)

Explanation: Sensitivity of the underlying disease to the allogeneic graft-versus-malignancy effect of DLI varies generally. Chronic myeloid leukaemia, myelofibrosis, and low-grade non-Hodgkin lymphoma and multiple myeloma show notably high sensitivity to DLI; chronic lymphocytic leukaemia, acute myeloid leukaemia, myelodysplastic syndrome, and Hodgkin lymphoma are considered to have intermediate sensitivity; and acute lymphoblastic leukaemia and diffuse large B-cell lymphoma, are considered to have a lower sensitivity to this therapeutic approach.

Q14. Ans(3)

Explanation: Dose escalation allows gradual immune activation, balancing GVL effects with acceptable GVHD risk. EBMT strongly supports this strategy across s disease setting as abrupt high dose DLI increases toxicity without improving outcome.

Q15. Ans(4)

Explanation: Delayed DLI allows partial immune tolerance and stabilization of host tissues. Studies shows that lower GVHD rates when DLI is administered later after HSCT. EBMT recommends a period of 90 days after the transplant for DLI (might be amended on the basis of type of donor, graft source, graft-versus host disease (GVHD) prophylaxis, and conditioning regimens).

Q16. Ans(1)

Explanation: Prophylactic DLIs are used as maintenance therapy for prevention of post-allogeneic HCT relapse, and are applied to patients without evidence of the underlying disease, who are estimated to bear a high risk of disease recurrence, based on one of three factors: high-risk disease characteristics (eg, unfavourable genetics or secondary disease); transplantation in refractory or advanced disease; and use of ex-vivo lymphocyte depletion as GVHD prophylaxis. Prophylactic DLIs can be considered in the case of non-myeloablative conditioning or in the absence of druggable molecular targets, irrespective of the conditioning regimen

Q17. Ans(2)

Explanation: EBMT recognizes haplo-DLI as feasible when lower initial doses and careful escalation are used. GVHD risk can be comparable to matched DLI when protocols are followed. It is no longer considered contra-indicated.

Q18. Ans(2)

Explanation: After DLI, close clinical and laboratory monitoring in the transplantation outpatient clinic is mandatory, considering all possible manifestations of GVHD and other side-effects. Serial monitoring of donor chimerism is important following DLI to assess the response status. Changes in chimerism often precede clinical remission or relapse. Other parameters have limited relevance in DLI setting.

Q19. Ans(3)

Explanation: EBMT highlights that [patients with predominant host haematopoiesis are at high risk for marrow aplasia after DLI. Rapid immune-mediated elimination of host cells may occur without adequate donor stem cell reserve.

Q20. Ans(3)

Explanation: Hydrocortisone should be avoided as it may blunt the GVT effect of DLI.

REFERENCES

1. Frederik Falkenburg JH, Schmid C, Kolb HJ, Kuball J. Delayed Transfer of Immune Cells or the Art of Donor Lymphocyte Infusion (DLI) 2.0. EBMT Handbook - HSCT and Cellular. Therapy. 2024;531–40.
2. Clinical applications of donor lymphocyte infusion from an HLA-haploidentical donor: consensus recommendations from the Acute Leukemia Working Party of the EBMT. Haematologica. 2020(1):47–58.
3. Cohn CS, Delaney M, Johnson ST, Katz LM, SchwartzJ, editors. Technical manual 21st ed. Washington, DC:AABB;2023

Chapter 14

CHIMERIC ANTIGEN RECEPTOR(CAR)-T THERAPY

Dr. Shahida and Dr. Swapna

Clinical History

Q1. A 10-month-old male patient diagnosed with acute lymphoblastic leukemia (pre-B ALL) has successfully completed his final chemotherapy treatment. Given his potential risk for relapse, the hematology/oncology team has requested the collection of peripheral blood chimeric antigen receptor (CAR) T-cells for possible salvage therapy and as a bridge to hematopoietic stem cell transplant (HSCT). The patient measures 60.7 cm in height and has a weight of 8.2 kg. His complete blood count (CBC) results are as follows: hemoglobin (Hgb) at 11.4 g/dL, hematocrit (Hct) at 33.8%, and a platelet count of 79 K/µL. Additionally, the patient's morning peripheral blood CD3 (T-cell) count is recorded at 542/µL.

A. Which of the following is false in CAR T-cell therapy?

1. It is a type of adoptive cellular immunotherapy
2. CARs are synthetic receptors that are utilized to genetically modify and reprogram T cells
3. Lentiviral vector transduction, which involves inserting the necessary genetic alterations using a virus, is used in modern CARs 4.None of the above

B. What are the indications of CAR T-cell therapy?

1. CAR T-cell therapy is used to treat relapsed or refractory multiple myeloma, acute lymphoblastic leukemias (ALL), and B-cell lymphomas (licensed by the USFDA)
2. Promising treatments for various hematological malignancies are being developed
3. CAR T-cell therapy treatments for solid tumors are also being developed
4. All of the above

C. What are the collection requirements for an effective CAR T-cell therapy?

1. Collection requirements are based on FDA-approved indications
2. *Tisagenlecleucel*, a CD19-directed immunotherapy (FDA-approved) is now the most well-known CAR T-cell therapy
3. A *total nucleated cell count of* 2.0×10^9 and a collection target dosage of 1.0×10^9 *CD3+* cells are required for the therapy
4. All of the above

D. What are the challenges expected with cellular collection in this small patient?

1. Peripheral venous access can be difficult
2. For a patient of this size; a *7-French double-lumen catheter* is recommended
3. This patient needs a *blood prime* in order to reduce the amount of extracorporeal blood required to fill the collection circuit
4. All of the above

E. What are the risks associated with cellular collection in this small patient?

1. There can be *30% decline* in the patient's estimated total blood volume (TBV)
2. The possibility of *blood clumping* during the collection is increased due to the slow speed
3. The patient's blood *calcium and occasionally magnesium* levels can drop
4. All of the above

F. What are the risks of administering CAR T-cell therapy?

1. The risks include *cytokine release syndrome* and *neurotoxicity* upon infusion of the manufactured cells
2. *Neutropenia, thrombocytopenia, and infections* are common complications
3. Failure of the infused CAR T cells to persist in vivo can also result in a *failed therapy* and there is also some potential for the engineered T cells to further *mutate*
4. All of the above

Q2. The defining structural component of a chimeric antigen receptor (CAR) that allows MHC-independent antigen recognition is the:
1. CD3ζ signalling domain
2. Costimulatory domain
3. Transmembrane domain
4. Single chain variable fragment

Q3. Which intracellular signalling domain is universally present in currently approved CAR-T constructs?
1. CD28
2. 4-1BB
3. CD3ζ
4. ICOS

Q4. The first clinically successful CAR-T therapies were directed against which antigens?
1. CD20
2. CD22
3. CD19
4. BCMA

Q5. Loss of CD19 expression following CAR-T therapy in ALL is most commonly due to:
1. Antibody neutralization
2. Alternative splicing or antigen escape
3. Complement mediated lysis
4. CAR-T exhaustion alone

Q6. Which strategy is currently explored to overcome antigen escape in CAR-T therapy?
1. Increasing lymphodepletion
2. Dual or bispecific CAR targeting
3. Higher CAR-T doses
4. Delayed infusion schedules

Q7. BCMA directed CATR-T cells are primarily used in the treatment of:
1. Acute lymphoblastic leukemia
2. Chronic lymphocytic leukemia
3. Hodgkin lymphoma
4. Multiple myeloma

Q8. The most common and predictable on-target/off-tumor toxicity of CD19 CAR-T therapy is:
1. CRS
2. Neurotoxicity
3. B cell aplasia
4. Capillary leak syndrome

Q9. The key cytokine driving cytokine release syndrome is:
1. IL-2
2. IFN-γ
3. TNF-α
4. IL-6

Q10. Which drug is first line therapy for severe CRS?
1. Corticosteroids
2. Rituximab
3. Cyclophosphamide
4. Tocilizumab

Q11. CAR-T therapy related neurotoxicity is best characterized by which feature?
1. IL-6 dependent and steroid responsive
2. Always associated with CNS leukemia
3. Poorly responsive to Tocilizumab
4. Due to CAR binding to neurons

Q12. High tumor burden prior to CAR-T cell infusion increases the risk of:

1. Graft rejection
2. CRS
3. CAR loss
4. Vector silencing

Q13. CAR-HEMATOTOX refers to:

1. Long lasting cytopenia after CAR-T
2. Hemolysis post infusion
3. Bone marrow fibrosis
4. Autoimmune pancytopenia

Q14. A major limitation of CAR-T therapy in solid tumor is:

1. Lack of T cell expansion
2. Absence of viral vectors
3. Immunosuppressive tumour microenvironment
4. Inability to engineer CARs

Q15. Unlike CARs, TCR- based therapies can recognize:

1. Only surface antigens
2. Intracellular antigens presented on MHCs
3. Glycolipids only
4. Soluble antigens

Q16. A MAJOR limitation of TCR-engineered therapies compared to CAR-T is:

1. Higher cost
2. MHC restriction
3. Lack of persistence
4. Limited expansion

Q17. Genome editing in CAR-T is primarily used to:

1. Increase immunogenicity
2. Knock out endogenous TCRs. 3. Prevent cytokine secretion
4. Reduce viral transduction

Q18. Targeted integration of CAR constructs into the TCR locus results in:

1. Reduced CAR expression
2. Improved long term expression
3. Increased immunogenicity
4. Loss of specificity

Q19. Which of the following is the promising alternative CAR in hematologic malignancies?

1. HER2
2. SLAMF7
3. EGFR
4. PSA

Q20. The future success of CAR-T therapy largely depends on all EXCEPT:

1. Identification of new targets
2. Improved genome editing tools
3. Elimination of lymphodepletion
4. Scalable GMP manufacturing

Q21. Core components of a CAR construct can include all except:

1. Antigen-binding domain
2. Transmembrane domain
3. Intra-cellular signalling domain
4. CD34 stem cell domain

Q22. CAR T cells recognize tumor antigens in a manner that is:
1. MHC class I restricted
2. MHC class II restricted
3. MHC independent
4. Antibody dependent only

Q23. CAR T cells used in current licensed products are MOST commonly derived from:
1. HLA-matched donor T cells
2. Umbilical cord blood lymphocytes
3. Autologous peripheral blood T cells
4. Bone marrow-derived lymphocytes

Q24. The PRIMARY purpose of lymphodepleting chemotherapy before CAR T infusion is to:
1. Reduce leukemia burden alone
2. Prevent cytokine release syndrome
3. Enhance CAR T expansion and persistence
4. Eliminate residual stem cells

Q25. Which CAR generation FIRST incorporated a costimulatory domain?
1. First generation CAR
2. Second generation CAR
3. Third generation CAR
4. Fourth generation CAR

Q26. Which FDA approved CAR T therapy targets multiple myeloma?
1. Axicabtagene ciloleucel
2. Tisagenlecleucel
3. Brexucabtagene autoleucel
4. Idecabtagene vicleucel

Q27. Which of the following is a universal "on target, off tumor" effect of CD19 CAR T therapy?
1. Pancytopenia
2. Hypogammaglobulinemia
3. Tumor lysis syndrome
4. Severe neutropenia

Q28. CAR-T therapy is currently MOST established for treatment of:
1. Solid tumors
2. Myeloid leukemia
3. Plasma cell leukemia
4. Relapsed/refractory B cell malignancies

Q29. Cytokine release syndrome CRS) is PRIMARILY mediated by:
1. Direct tumor lysis
2. Excessive cytokine secretion by activated immune cells
3. Complement activation
4. Antibody-dependent cytotoxicity

Q30. Immune effector cell-associated neurotoxixty syndrome (ICANS) is MOST closely associated with:
1. CAR-T cell trafficking to CNS
2. Blood-barrier disruption due to cytokines
3. Direct neuronal CAR binding
4. Viral vector neurotoxicity

Q31. Loss of CD19 expression following CAR-T therapy MOST commonly results in:
1. GVHD
2. Treatment related mortality
3. Antigen-negative relapse
4. Manufacturing failure

Q32. Which factor MOST strongly correlates with the severity of CRS?
1. Patient age
2. Prior lines of therapy
3. Tumour burden at infusion
4. Viral vector type

Q33. Which CAR design feature MOST improves long-term CAR-T persistence?
1. High-affinity scFv alone
2. Inclusion of a costimulatory domain
3. Shortened transmembrane domain
4. Removal of signalling domain

Q34. Compared with CD28-based CARs, 4-IBB-based Cars are associated with:
1. Faster expansion but shorter persistence
2. Slower expansion but longer persistence
3. Higher CRS severity
4. Universal neurotoxicity

Q35. Bridging therapy before CAR-T infusion is used PRIMARILLY to:
1. Prevent CRS
2. Improve CAR-T manufacturing
3. Control disease while CAR-T cells are prepared
4. Enhance lymphodepletion

Q36. Which long term complication requires ongoing monitoring after CAR-T therapy?
1. Iron overload
2. Hypogammaglobulinemia
3. Hemochromatosis
4. Secondary polycythaemia

Q37. Strategies to overcome antigen escape include all EXCEPT
1. Dual-target CARs
2. Sequential CAR-T infusions
3. Targeting alternative antigens
4. Avoiding lymphodepletion

Q38. Factors influencing CRS severity include:
1. Tumour burden
2. CAR-T expansion
3. Baseline inflammation
4. ABO blood group

Q39. Which CAR-T modification improves safety by enabling selective elimination of CAR-T cells?
1. Dual CARs
2. Suicide gene incorporation
3. Armored CARs
4. Affinity tuning

Q40. Which immune cell population contributes significantly to CRS amplification?
1. Neutrophils
2. Eosinophils
3. Macrophages
4. Platelets

Q41. Which feature most distinguishes 3rd generation CARs from 2nd generation CARs?
1. Absence of CD3ζ
2. Two costimulatory domains
3. Antibody based recognition
4. Use of non-viral vectors

Q42. Which premedication to be avoided in CAR-T cell expansion?

1. Chlorpheniramine
2. Hydrocortisone
3. Acetaminophen
4. Antipyretics

Q43. After thawing, CAR-T product in cryobags is stable at room temperature for:

1. 4 to 6 hours
2. 24 hours
3. 30 to 3 hours
4. 12 hours

Q44. During infusion, the following things are to be taken care of:

1. Spiked using DMSO resistant spikes
2. Infused using a standard blood transfusion set
3. Leukocyte reduction filter should never be used
4. Should not be irradiated

Choose the right answer from the given options:

1. 1, 2 and 3 are correct
2. 1 and 3 are correct
3. 2 and 4 are correct
4. all are correct

Q45. Toxicities following CAR-T cell therapy include:

1. Macrophage activation syndrome
2. Acute graft versus host disease
3. Tumor lysis syndrome
4. Malignant transformation of CAR-T cells

Choose the right answer from the given options:

1. 1,2,3 are correct
2. 1,3,4 are correct
3. 2,4 are correct
4. all are correct

Q46. The FDA has approved the following CAR-T cell formulations for large B cell lymphoma except:

1. Lisocabtagene maraleucel
2. Tisagenlecleucel
3. Ciltacabtagene autoleucel
4. Axicabtageneciloleucel

Q47. On target, off tumor effects of CAR-T cell therapy due to target expression on the benign tissue can be reduced with all the following approaches except:

1. Affinity tuning of the receptor
2. Transient receptor expression
3. Regional cell delivery
4. Epitope spreading

Q48. All are gene editing techniques used in allogenic CAR-T cell preparation EXCEPT:

1. Zinc finger nuclease
2. Transcription activator-like effector nuclease
3. CRISPR/Cas9 platforms
4. HSV-TK gene insertion

Q49. CAR-T cell therapy requires long-term follow-up PRIMARILY to monitor for:

1. Iron overload
2. Insertional oncogenesis
3. Secondary hemoglobinopathies
4. Autoimmune cytopenias

ANSWERS

Q1. A. Ans(4)

Explanation: Adoptive transfer of ex-vivo modified immune cells is a component of CAR-T cell therapy. One treatment approach that potentially uses the body's own innate and adaptive immune response to cancer is cell-based immunotherapy. It is not the same as immune checkpoint inhibitors or passive antibody treatments.

B. Ans(4)
C. Ans(4)
D. Ans(4)
E. Ans(4)
F. Ans(4)

Q2. Ans(4)

Explanation: CARs detect target antigens independently of MHC through an extracellular Single chain variable fragment (scFv), which is derived from the variable regions of mononuclear antibodies. This design allows CAR-T cells to directly engage surface antigens on the tumor cells. In contrast to T cell receptors (TCRs), CARs do not rely on antigen processing or presentation by MHC molecules.

Q3. Ans(3)

Explanation: The CD3ζ signalling domain is a fundamental component of all CARconstructs and is responsible for delivering the primary activation signal upon antigen engagement. While costimulatory domains such as CD28 or 4-1BBenhance T cell expansion and long term persistence, they are not present in every design. CD3ζ remains indispensable for initiating T-cell activation.

Q4. Ans(3)

Explanation: CD19 was the first antigen effectively targeted by CAR-T cells, demonstrating lasting complete remissions in refractory B cell malignancies. Its reliable expression on B-lineage cells rendered it an optimal initial target. These outcomes facilitated the path for regulatory approvals.

Q5. Ans(2)

Explanation: Resistance to CAR-T therapy frequently arises from antigen escape mechanisms. Tumor cells may undergo alternative splicing, lineage switching, or selective expansion of CD19-negative clones, thereby evading CAR recognition. Such antigen loss variants represent a major cause of relapse and continue to pose a significant therapeutic challenge.

Q6. Ans(2)

Explanation: Dual or bispecific CARs are engineered to recognize two target antigens simultaneously, thereby reducing the risk of tumor escape. This can be accomplished using tandem CAR constructs containing two scFvs within a single receptor or through co-expression of separate CAR molecules in the same T cell. Such approaches aim to improve durability of response. Current research is evaluating combinations such as CD19 with either CD20, CD22, or CD123 using both cis-configured bispecific CARs and dual CAR expression approaches to enhance response durability.

Q7. Ans(4)

Explanation: B-cell maturation antigen (BCMA) is selectively expressed on plasma cells, making it an ideal therapeutic target in multiple myeloma. BCMA directed CAR- T products have demonstrated high response rates and have received regulatory approval. Plasma cell aplasia is an anticipated on-target effect, leading to hypogammaglobulinemia due to depletion of antibody producing cells, necessitating ongoing immunoglobulin replacement therapy.

Q8. Ans(3)

Explanation: The most predictable toxicity of CAR-T therapy is the depletion of normal cells expressing the target antigen. For example, infusion of CD-19directed CAR-T cells in ALL, NHL, and CLL patients have resulted in prolonged B-cell aplasia because CD19 is expressed on healthy B cells. This leads to hypogammaglobinaemia requiring immunoglobulin replacement and serve as evidence of effective biological activity.

Q9. Ans(4)

Explanation: CRS is seen when CAR-T-cell recognize tumour cells, resulting in massive release of massive inflammatory cytokines, often amplified by activation of innate immune cells. IL-6 plays a pivotal role in CRS pathogenesis. Therapeutic blockade of the IL-6 receptor with Tocilizumab frequently results in rapid clinical improvement, highlighting that IL-6 as the central mediator of this toxicity.

Q10. Ans(4)

Explanation: Tocilizumab, an anti-IL-6 receptor monoclonal antibody, is the standard first line treatment for severe form of CRS. It rapidly reverses fever and hemodynamic instability. Corticosteroids are reserved for refractory cases.

Q11. Ans(3)

Explanation: Neurotoxicity associated with CAR-T cell therapies is often unresponsive to Tocilizumab, suggesting mechanism beyond IL-6. It can occur without CNS disease involvement. Severe case may lead to cerebral edema and death.

Q12. Ans(2)

Explanation: Patients with a high tumour burden experience more intense CAR-T activation, increasing cytokine release. This correlates with a higher incidence and severity of CRS. Tumour burden is an important risk-stratification factor.

Q13. Ans(1)

Explanation: CAR-HEMATOTX describes prolonged cytopenia following CAR-T therapy, associated with increased infection risk. The exact mechanism remains unclear but is clinically significant. Supportive care and monitoring are essential.

Q14. Ans(3)
Explanation: Application of CAR-T therapy to solid tumours is limited by several obstacles, including antigen heterogeneity, difficult accessibility, poor trafficking, and immunosuppressive microenvironments. These barriers reduce CAR-T efficacy in solid tumours compared to hematologic malignancies. Innovative CAR designs and combinational strategies are being developed to address these limitations.

Q15. Ans(2)
Explanation: Unlike CARs that recognize only surface antigens, TCRs. identify peptide fragments derived from intracellular proteins that are presented by MHC molecules. This enables targeting of tumour-specific intracellular antigens, including many oncogenic driver mutations. Since most of the tumour-specific or tumour-associated antigens are intracellular, they are accessible to TCR-based therapies, but not to CAR-T cells, which remain restricted to surface targets.

Q16. Ans(2)
Explanation: TCR based therapies are limited by HLA restriction, requiring the development of distinct TCR constructs for different HLA types. This constraint reduces its broad applicability. Thus, to provide TCR therapy across diverse patient populations, multiple antigen-specific TCRs. must be generated for various HLA alleles. In contrast, CAR-T cell therapy circumvents this issue through MHC independent antigen recognition.

Q17. Ans(2)
Explanation: Genome editing can eliminate the endogenous TCR to enhance expression of the introduced transgenic receptor and reduce the risk of TCR chain mispairing, which may cause autoreactive T-cells. Gene editing techniques such as CRISPR/Car9 improve product safety, promote uniform CAR expression and are essential for developing allogenic "off-the-shelf" cellular therapies.

Q18. Ans(2)
Explanation: Insertion of the CAR construct into the endogenous TCR locus allows regulated and sustained receptor expression. This approach enhances persistence and functional stability while reducing variability associated with random genomic integration. Such precision engineering may improve long-term therapeutic outcomes.

Q19. Ans(2)
Explanation: Approved cellular therapies are now being evaluated earlier in the treatment algorithms, and substantial efforts are underway to identify additional CAR targets hematologic malignancies. Emerging targets include SLAMF7, CD44v6, CD38, CD33, CD70, CD123, CLL-1, and FLT3. For example, SLAMF7 is expressed in multiple myeloma and other hematologic malignancies and is underactive investigation. Expanding the target selection broadens the therapeutic scope beyond CD19 and BCMA.

Q20. Ans(3)
Explanation: Lymphodepleting chemotherapy remains essential CAR-T cell therapy to facilitate optimal T-cell expansion and persistence. Future innovations are focused on refining antigen targets, advancing gene-editing techniques, and improving scalable manufacturing processes. Complete elimination of lymphodepletion is unlikely in the foreseeable future.

Q21. Ans(4)
Explanation: CD34 stem cell domain is not a part of CAR-T cell construct. A CAR is a synthetic molecule which is composed of an extracellular antigen-recognition domain, a transmembrane segment, and intracellular signalling domains for T cell activation. The antigen recognition domain is made from antigen- binding portion of an antibody that recognizes cancer cell target antigen. On binding with the antigen, the intracellular signalling machinery of a TCR complex is activated enabling the CAR T cells to undergo multiplication.

Q22. Ans(3)
Explanation: CAR-T cells recognizes cancer cell target antigen through the antibody derived binding region. The concept behind CAR T cells is to exploit the antigen-recognition properties of antibodies with the effector (killing) ability of T cells. CAR-T cells recognize antigens independently of MHC molecules because the antigen-binding domain is derived from antibodies. This allows CAR T cells to overcome tumour immune evasion due to MHC down-regulation. This feature is a major advantage over conventional T cell response.

Q23. Ans(3)
Explanation: Most commercially approved CAR T therapies use autologous peripheral blood T cells collected by leukapheresis. This avoids the risk of graft versus host diseases and graft rejection. Allogenic CAR T products remains largely investigational.

Q24. Ans(3)
Explanation: Lymphodepletion reduces endogenous competing lymphocytes and increases homeostatic cytokines such as IL-7 and IL-15. This promotes CAR T cell expansion and persistence after infusion. It is a critical preparative step for therapeutic efficiency.

Q25. Ans(2)
Explanation: First- generation CARs connect the scFv to CD3ζ chain which is the signal-transduction molecule of T- cell antigen receptor. However, first generation CARS showed limited clinical efficacy with reduced persistence. This poor persistence was due to the absence of co-stimulation. Thus, second generation CARs were generated by the addition of one costimulatory domain like CD28 or 4-IBB alongside CD3ζ. This innovation markedly improved T cell activation and persistence.

Q26. Ans(4)
Explanation: Idacabtagene vicleucel targets BCMA and is approved for relapsed/refractory multiple myeloma. Other listed products target CD19 in B cell malignancies.

Q27. Ans(2)
Explanation: As CD-19 expressed on both benign and malignant B-cells, CD-19 directed CAR-T cell therapy can bind to normal and the tumour cells. Thus, CD-19 cell ablation by the CD19 directed CART-cells lead to the loss of entire B-cell compartment resulting in B- cell aplasia. It may necessitates Immunoglobulin replacement therapy though its use controversial.

Q28. Ans(4)
Explanation: CAR T-cells have demonstrated strongest clinical efficacy for treating refractory relapsed B- cell leukemias compared to CAR T- cell response for multiple myeloma, B- cell lymphoma, and other hematologic malignancies. B- cell maturation antigen (BCMA)- directed CAR T-cells have shown 73% overall response in patients with refractory/relapsed multiple myeloma whereas CD19 directed CAR T-cells have shown around 50% response rates in patients with B- cell lymphomas. Efficacy rate in solid tumours is limited due to tumour microenvironment barriers and antigen heterogeneity.

Q29. Ans(2)
Explanation: CRS is characterized by an immune-mediated production of excessive inflammatory markers and cytokines, leading to a positive feedback loop of immune hyperactivation. The pathogenesis involves a complicated interplay between host macrophages and CAR-T cells. Activated CAR-T cells directly kill all target-positive cells, along with secretion of several proinflammatory cytokines including IFNγ, IL-1, IL-5, IL-6, IL-10, IL-2-receptor alpha, GM-CSF and nitric oxide. Signs and symptoms of CRS include fever, fatigue, myalgias, head ache, hypotension, tachycardia, coagulopathy, hypoxia, and multiple organ failure. The severity of CRS correlates with tumour burden and CAR-T expansion.

Q30. Ans(2)
Explanation: ICANS commonly overlaps with CRS; however, it may also develop at different phase of treatment. Further, ICANS has been reported with CAR-T products targeting antigens other than CD19, indicating that its occurrence is not dependent on the specific target antigen. In ICANS, current evidence shows that excessive immune activation results in endothelial dysfunction and disruption of the blood brain barrier. This increased permeability allows inflammatory mediators and immune cells to enter the central nervous system, where escalating neuroinflammation produces neurological manifestations. Notably, CAR-T cells are not consistently detected in the CSF of affected patients, implying that host immune mechanisms play a significant role in ICANS pathogenesis. There is no evidence that CAR-T cells exert direct cytotoxic effects on neurons.

Q31. Ans(3)
Explanation: Relapse following CAR-T cell therapy can occur due to antigen escape, most commonly through deletion or mutation of the CD19 antigen. In some cases, insertion of the CAR construct during transduction alters the leukemic cell genome, leading to loss or modification of the CD19 epitope that is required for CAR recognition. As a result, malignant cells evade immune targeting. These observations underscore the importance of developing CAR-T strategies that simultaneously targets multiple antigens to minimize relapse.

Q32. Ans(3)
Explanation: Explanation: An increased disease or tumour burden prior to the treatment is associated with heightened CAR-T cell activation and amplified cytokine production. Consequently, patients with high tumour load are at greater risk of developing severe CRS. Additional factors that contribute to increased CRS severity include administration of large CAR-T cell dose, prior lymphodepletion using fludarabine based regimens, and pre-existing clinical states characterized by elevated inflammatory cytokines. In contrast, patient's age and the type of viral vectors used for CAR construct have a comparatively limited impact.

Q33. Ans(2)
Explanation: Incorporation of costimulatory signalling domains such as CD28 or 4-IBBinto CAR construct significantly improves T cell expansion, survival and in vivo persistence, representing a key advancement over first generation CAR designs. Comparative studies have demonstrated superior proliferation and durability of cytotoxic T lymphocytes engineered with CD-28 based co stimulation. Sustained persistence of CAR-T cells is a critical determinant of long-term disease control and durable remission.

Q34. Ans(2)
Explanation: CAR-T cells incorporating 4-1BB costimulatory domains typically show slower early expansion but demonstrate enhanced long-term persistence. In contrast, CD28-based CARs undergo rapid proliferation but tend to persist for shorter periods. CD28, belonging to the immunoglobulin superfamily, serves as central co-stimulatory receptor that enhances T cell activation by driving metabolic programming toward glycolysis. This metabolic shift supports the biosynthetic demands of rapid cell division and effector activity. Conversely, 4-1BB signalling, a member of the tumour necrosis factor receptor family, favours mitochondrial oxidative phosphorylation and promotes differentiation toward a central memory phenotype. Enhanced mitochondrial function and biogenesis are associated with improved antitumor efficacy, and CAR-T cells with 4-1BB co-stimulation have been shown to persists in patients for over a decade.

Q35. Ans(3)

Explanation: Bridging therapy is used to stabilize or reduce rapidly progressive diseases while CAR-T cells are being manufactured. Its role is limited to diseases control during this interval and it neither substitutes for lymphodepleting chemotherapy nor directly reduces the risk of CRS.

Q36. Ans(2)

Explanation: Following CD19 directed CAR-T therapy, sustained B cell aplasia commonly results in prolonged hypogammaglobulinemia. Affected patients often require long-term immunoglobulin replacement and careful surveillance for infections. This represents a well-recognized and expected delayed complication of CAR-T cell therapy.

Q37. Ans(4)

Explanation: Targeting multiple tumour antigens reduces the likelihood of relapse caused by antigen loss or modulation. Many cellular immunotherapy protocols rely on supportive treatments, such as lymphodepleting chemotherapy with agents like fludarabine, to optimize CAR-T cell expansion and function. Although these drugs are not components of the final cellular product, they may be essential elements of the overall testament regimen.

Q38. Ans(4)

Explanation: The likelihood of developing severe CRS is increased in patients with a high tumour burden prior to therapy, those receiving larger CAR-T cell doses, individuals treated with fludarabine based lymphodepletion, and patients with elevated baseline inflammatory cytokines. In contrast, ABO blood group does not influence CRS risk.

Q39. Ans(2)

Explanation: Safety mechanisms like suicide genes enable selective elimination of CAR-T cells if life threatening toxicity develops. These inducible systems allow termination of CAR-T cell activity without negating initial therapeutic benefit. One such approach involves pro-drugs like ganciclovir, which remains inactive until phosphorylated by herpes simplex virus thymidine kinase (HSV-TK). CAR-T cell engineered to express HSV-TK can therefore be selectively destroyed upon ganciclovir exposure, offering a method for in vivo control of toxicity.

Q40. Ans(3)

Explanation: CRS arises from a complex interaction between infused Car- T cells and host immune cells, particularly macrophages. Activated CAR-T cells eradicate antigen-positive targets while simultaneously releasing proinflammatory cytokines. CRS is characterized by elevated levels of multiple mediators, including IFN-γ, IL-1, IL-6, IL-10, GM-CSF, IL-5, IL-2 receptor alpha, and nitric oxide. GM-CSF secretion and CD40Lexpression on CAR-T cells promote recruitment, activation, and expansion of endogenous macrophages, which are major sources of IL-1, IL-6 and IFN-γ. These activated macrophages perpetuate a cytokine amplification loop, resulting in the systemic hyperinflammatory manifestations typical of CRS.

Q41. Ans(2)

Explanation: While second generation autologous CAR-T cells can induce rapid remissions and serve as a bridge to a curative transplantation, the emergence of cancer cells with antigen evasion (antigen escape) and limited cellular persistence remains significant challenges. Moreover, long-term persistence of CAR-T cells is essential for durable clinical remissions. These limitations resulted in the development of third generation CARs which incorporated two co-stimulatory domains which combined CD28 and 4-1BB signalling domains.

Q42. Ans(2)

Explanation: CAR-T cell infusion is generally performed several days after completion of the conditioning regimen. Pre-medications are administered to reduce infusion related reactions and typically include an H1 antihistamine, such as diphenhydramine, and an antipyretic, such as Acetaminophen, given 30-60 minutes beforehand. Prophylactic corticosteroids are avoided, as they may impair CAR-T cell expansion and function.

Q43. Ans(3)

Explanation: After thawing, CAR-T cells products remain stable at room temperature (20-25 C) for a manufacture-specified duration. This window varies by product, ranging from 30 minutes for tisagenlecleucel (Kymriah) to up to 3hours for products such as Axicabtagene ciloleucel or Brexucabtagene autolecleucel (Yescarta/Tecartus). Topreserve optimal cell viability and efficacy, the interval between thawing and infusion should be kept as short as possible.

Q44. Ans(4)

Administration of CAR-T cells closely resembles standard stem cell infusion procedures. Because DMSO is commonly used as cryoprotectant, all tubing and spikes must be compatible with DMSO. A conventional blood filter (150-260 µm) may be used; however, leukocyte reduction filters must be avoided and the cellular product should never be irradiated.

Q45. Ans(2)

Explanation: Beyond CRS and ICANS, CAR- T cell therapy may be associated with other adverse effects, including macrophage activation syndrome, prolonged cytopenias, infections, and tumour lysis syndrome. As CAR-T therapy involves permanent genetic modification using viral vectors, there is a theoretical risk of malignant transformation. Consequently, the FDA mandated long-term follow-up of treated patients for up to 15 years after infusion.

Q46. Ans(3)

Currently, six CAR-T cell therapies have received FDA approval for hematologic malignancies: idecabtagene vicleucel and ciltacabtagene autoleucel for multiple myeloma, lisocabtagene maraleucel, axicabtageneciloleucel and tisagenlecleucel for large B-cell lymphoma; brexucabtagene autoleucel for mantle cell lymphoma; and, axicabtageneciloleucel additionally for acute lymphoblastic leukaemia.

Q47. Ans(4)

Explanation: Expression of target antigens on normal tissues, even at low levels, poses a significant risk for "on target, off tumour" effects. Several strategies have been developed to mitigate this risk, including receptor affinity tuning, transient CAR expression, and regional delivery of CAR-T cells. Affinity-tuned CARs are designed to recognize antigens only above a defined density threshold, enabling effective tumour killing while sparing normal tissues with low antigen expression. Alternatively, CART cells can be generated using CAR mRNA, resulting in temporary target receptor expression. Lastly, regional or intra tumoral administration of cellular immunotherapy may further confine the inflammatory response to the tumour site and limit effects on distant benign tissue.

Epitope spreading represents another off-target phenomenon of CAR-T cell therapy, whereby tumour cell destruction released additional antigens in a proinflammatory environment. These antigens are processed by antigen presenting cells and presented to the naïve T cells, potentially broadening the immune response beyond the originally targeted epitope.

Q48. Ans(4)

Explanation: Allogeneic CAR-T cell approaches may address many limitations of autologous therapies, such as insufficient T-cell numbers, impaired T cell quality, or contamination of the apheresis product with many non-T cells. However, donor derived CAR-T cells introduce distinct risks, as their native HLA molecules can rigger immune rejection by the recipient. More critically, expression of an alloreactive endogenous T-cell receptor may result in severe graft versus host disease. Gene-editing technologies can mitigate these risks by disrupting the HLA/and /or TCR expression. Platforms such as Zinc finger nuclease, transcription activator-like effector nuclease (TALENs), and CRISPR/Cas9 have been developed for precise editing of HLA and TCR loci.

Q49. Ans(2)

Explanation: CAR-T cell therapies relies on genetic modification of T-cells using viral vectors or nucleic acids to integrate the CAR transgene into the host genome. While genomic integration enables sustained transgene expression throughout the lifespan of the cell, it also introduces potential risks. These include insertional mutagenesis leading to malignant transformation (Insertional oncogenesis) or other mutations (Insertional mutagenesis) with negative consequences. Although malignant transformation has not been reported, non-oncogenic insertional effects may still have adverse consequences. One reported case involved a patient with B-cell ALL who relapsed after an initial complete remission; analysis revealed that CAR integration disrupted the CD19expression in the leukemic cells, rendering them invisible to the CAR-T cells. This case highlights a serious, albeit rare, complication associated with the genetic engineering process inherent to CAR-T cell therapy.

REFERENCES

1. Zhang H, Zhao P, Huang H. Engineering better chimeric antigen receptor T cells. Exp Hematol Oncol. 2020;9:34.
2. Feins S, Kong W, Williams EF, Milone MC, Fraietta JA. An introduction to chimeric antigen receptor (CAR) T-cell immunotherapy for human cancer. Am J Hematol. 2019;94(S1):S3–9.
3. Holmes B. CAR T-cell therapy indications grow significantly in 2021. Targeted Ther Oncol. 2021;10(8):10.
4. Cohn CS, Delaney M, Johnson ST, Katz LM, SchwartzJ, editors. Technical manual 21st ed. Washington, DC:AABB;2023
5. Neelapu SS, Locke FL, Bartlett NL, Lekakis LJ, Miklos DB, Jacobson CA, et al. Axicabtagene ciloleucel CAR T-cell therapy in refractory large B-cell lymphoma. N Engl J Med. 2017;377(26):2531–44.
6. Lana MG, Strauss BE. Production of lentivirus for the establishment of CAR-T cells. Methods Mol Biol. 2020;2086:61–7.
7. Allen ES, Stroncek DF, Ren J, Eder AF, West KA, Fry TJ, et al. Autologous lymphapheresis for the production of chimeric antigen receptor T cells. Transfusion. 2017;57(5):1133–41.
8. M. T. Friedman et al., "CAR T"-esian Thinking. *Immunohematology, Transfusion Medicine, Hemostasis, and Cellular Therapy Springer Nature Switzerland AG 2023.*
9. Raffaella Greco and Dominique Farge. CART Cells and Other Cell Therapies (ie MSC, Tregs) in Autoimmune Diseases. EBMT Handbook – HSCT and Cellular Therapy 2024; p837-48.
10. Andrew D. Fesnak and Don L. Siegel. Chimeric antigen receptor T cells and other cellular immunotherapies. Rossi's Principles of Transfusion Medicine. 6 th Edn. John Wiley & Sons Ltd. 2022; p633-41.
11. Cook MS, King E, Flaherty KR, Siddika K, Papa S, Benjamin R, et al. CAR-T cells containing CD28 versus 4-1BB co-stimulatory domains show distinct metabolic profiles in patients. Cell Rep [Internet]. 2025;44(7):115973. Available from: http://dx.doi.org/10.1016/j.celrep.2025.115973

Chapter 15

GRANULOCYTES

Dr. Sunantha

Q1. Which of the following is generally is not considered as an indication of granulocyte transfusion?

1. Severe neutropenia (ANC <0.5 × 10^9/L due to congenital or acquired bone marrow failure syndromes)
2. Receiving active treatment to achieve disease remission
3. Fungal or bacterial infection which is unresponsive to appropriate antimicrobial therapy
4. Pyrexia of unknown origin (PUO)

Q2. Which of the following could be a potential indication of granulocyte transfusion?

1. Viral infection (in absence of fungal or bacterial infection) and when patients are unresponsive to appropriate antimicrobial therapy
2. Sepsis (accompanied with absence of neutropenia)
3. Patients suffering from bone marrow failure where neutrophil recovery is not expected to recur spontaneously
4. Patients where neutrophil recovery is expected soon (weeks time)

Q3. Which of the following is true regarding natural G-CSF?

1. Granulocyte colony-stimulating factor (G-CSF), a protein that stimulates the growth of new blood cells
2. It was isolated from human cells by Malcolm Moore and Karl Welte in 1984
3. G-CSF mainly stimulates the myeloid cell series from committed progenitor cells to mature neutrophil granulocytes
4. All of the above

Q4. Which of the following is false regarding natural G-CSF?

1. Human G-CSF (hG-CSF) is located on chromosome 17 and encoded by CSF3 gene; and in healthy individuals, G-CSF levels are normally not measurable as it is below 100 pg/ml
2. The G-CSF b (174 amino acids) contains a glycosylation site on the oxygen known as O- linked glycosylation
3. Effects of G-CSF are mediated by binding to a single homodimer receptor, granulocyte colony stimulating factor receptor (G-CSFR)
4. None of the above

Q5. Which of the following is false regarding the transit time of neutrophils?

1. G-CSF expands the marrow neutrophil mitotic pool and it also shortens the transit time of differentiating neutrophils through the postmitotic pool
2. Following G-CSF injection, the postmitotic transit time in healthy volunteers decreases from 6.4 days to 2.9days
3. In vitro, the entire transit period from myeloblast to mature neutrophil is ten to twelve days
4. None of the above

Q6. Which of the following is true regarding mobilization of neutrophils?

1. The storage pool consists of mature neutrophils that remain in bone marrow for 4–6 days and responds to microbial invaders
2. The neutrophils baseline is estimated at 4.4 × 10^9/L, with 0.87 × 10^9 cells/kg released every day into the circulation
3. About 2% of neutrophils circulate in the bloodstream (90% retained in the bone marrow) and the half-life of neutrophils in circulation is 6–8 hours
4. All of the above

Q7. Identify the scientist

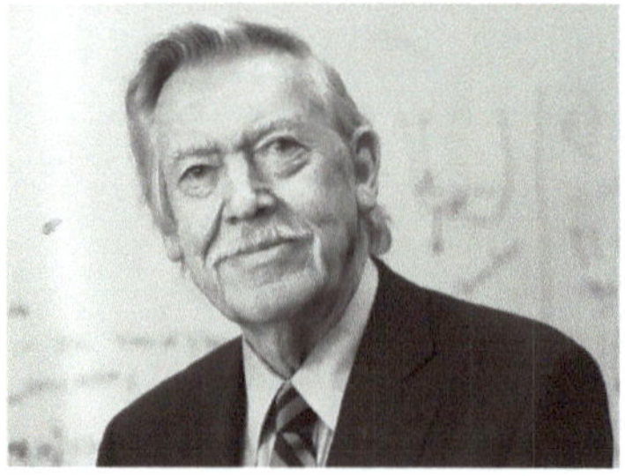

Fig-XIII-1: Reproduced from Welte K, Mertelsmann R. (13) 2025 Licensed under Creative Commons Attribution 4.0 International (CC BY 4.0). Image description given in answer key

1. R. Schofield
2. Thomas E Donall
3. Dr. Christian Barnard
4. Malcolm A.S.Moore

Q8. Which of the following is true regarding neutrophil receptor?

1. The retention, mobilization, and homing of neutrophils to and from the bone marrow are regulated by molecular mechanisms involving CXCR4 (C-X-C motif receptor 4), CXCR2 (C-X-C motif receptor 2), and CXCL12 (C-X-C motif ligand 12)
2. CXCR4 is a cytokine receptor important for the *homing* of stem cells and more mature neutrophils to the bone marrow and also to *maintain* neutrophils in the bone marrow, whereas CXCR2 is necessary for their *release*
3. A mutation in CXCR4 resulting enhanced responsiveness to CXCL12 underlies the WHIM syndrome
4. All of the above

Q9. Which of the following is true regarding the studies conducted on granulocyte transfusions?

1. Hester et al. came out reported an outcome of 60% (9 of 15) success with fungus (11 patients) and yeast (4 patients) using G-CSF 5 μg/kg stimulation
2. Price et al. reported an outcome of 100% (4 of 4) success with bacterial infection and 57% with yeast infection using both G-CSF (600 μg/kg) and dexamethasone (8 mg)
3. Lee at al. came out reported an outcome of 40% (10 of 25) success with multiple organism infections
4. All of the above

Q10. Which of the following is true regarding the donor screening for granulocyte donation?

1. Granulocyte donor should meet the same standards as per the blood donor screening standards
2. If the recipient is CMV negative; screening CMV negative donors should be considered
3. Before starting steroids, a proper history of hypertension, diabetes, cataracts, or peptic ulcer is mandatory
4. All of the above

Q11. Which of the following is false regarding the donor screening for granulocyte donation?

1. Complete blood count with Hemoglobin 12.5 gm/dl minimum, WBC counts within the normal range and normal platelet count
2. Assessment of renal function and liver function for the use of HES
3. HLA antigen profile similarity between donor and recipient
4. None of the above

Q12. Which of the following is true regarding the donation interval of granulocyte donation by apheresis?

1. Gap between two donations by apheresis is 3 months
2. A donor can donate up to four times a year unstimulated
3. A donor can be mobilized once a year up to a maximum of 4 times in a lifetime
4. All of the above

Q13. Which of the following is false regarding the donation interval of granulocyte donation by apheresis?

1. Gap between granulocyte apheresis and platelet apheresis is 30 days
2. If the reinfusion is incomplete then the donor is deferred for 90 days (male donors)
3. If the reinfusion is incomplete then the donor is deferred for 120 days (female donors)
4. None of the above

Q14. Which of the following is true regarding the medication for mobilization of the granulocyte donor?

1. 8 mg oral dexamethasone 12 hours before the donation
2. 60 mg oral dexamethasone at 2 hours before the donation
3. G-CSF 5-10 microgram/kg given 12 hours before collection
4. All of the above

Q15. Which of the following is true regarding the mobilization of the granulocyte donor?

1. Corticosteroids stimulation results in 2-3 times of the absolute neutrophil counts with a peak at 24 hours
2. G-CSF stimulation results in 7-10 times increase in the absolute neutrophil counts with a peak at 12 hours
3. G-CSF with corticosteroid stimulation results in 10-13.5 times increase in absolute neutrophil counts with a peak 12 hours.
4. All of the above

Q16. Which of the following is true with respect to Hydroxy ethyl starch

1. Granulocytes can be efficiently collected by using a combination of 6% HES (Medium Molecular Weight, MMW) and 46.7% trisodium citrate
2. HES (MMW) along with trisodium citrate is extremely safe and citrate toxicity can be avoided as ACD is not used
3. HighMolecularWeight-HES can give potential risks to healthy donors (kidney failures, bleeding disorders and impairment of hematopoiesis)
4. All of the above

Q17. Which of the following is true regarding the metabolism of Hydroxy ethyl starch HES?

1. HES is distributed to the interstitial tissue, which serves as a secondary compartment for prolonged deposition
2. In contrast to single apheresis, multiple apheresis results in the accumulation of HES within interstitial tissues due to its two-compartment distribution
3. HES is rapidly metabolized by the kidneys and eliminated through urine
4. All of the above

Q18. Which of the following is true regarding the side effects of HES?

1. HES can lead to acute kidney injury
2. HES disturbs the blood coagulation mechanism and hence increases the risk of bleeding
3. The immunomodulatory characteristics of HES influence the defence mechanisms of the body making them prone to infections, present with skin rashes to severe anaphylactic reactions
4. All of the above

Q19. Which of the following is true regarding Modified Fluid Gelatin (MFG)?

1. MFG has a biological half-life of 2.5 h in the body
2. It has enhanced renal clearance compared to HES
3. Granulocyte yields seem to be lower with MFG
4. All of the above

Q20. Which of the following is true regarding the dosage of granulocyte transfusion?

1. Doses of at least 1×10^{10} granulocytes per transfusion are required to treat or prevent infection
2. Neonates are transfused at a rate of 10-15 ml/kg (final dose of $1\text{-}2 \times 10^9$ granulocytes/kg per dose)
3. Transfusion can continue until the absolute neutrophil count is $>1.0 \times 10^9$/L on 2 consecutive days
4. All of the above

Q21. Which of the following is not true regarding the storage and transport of granulocytes?

1. TA- GVHD is prevented by irradiation with a dose of 25 Gray
2. Storage at 20-24 deg Celsius ideally without agitation
3. Shelf life is 5 days
4. It should not be transported via pneumatic tube

Q22. Which of the following is false regarding quality control regarding of granulocytes according to DGHS guidelines?

1. Volume: 200-400 ml
2. Concentration: 1×10^{10} granulocytes
3. Hematocrit: 50%±5%
4. None of the above

Q23. Which of the following is not true regarding granulocyte transfusion?
1. Always irradiate the product
2. The whole dose should be infused over 1-2 hours
3. Always leukodeplete the product
4. Granulocytes should be transfused through a standard red cell transfusion set.

Q24. Which of the following is NOT true about Adverse transfusion reaction related to Granulocyte transfusion?
1. The granulocyte concentrate contains a significant amount of lymphocyte contamination, which inherently increases the risk of TA-GvHD
2. Granulocytes present recipients with extra donor HLA antigens, potentially leading to HLA alloimmunization
3. Chills, fever and/or slight alterations in blood pressure
4. A syndrome similar to transfusion-associated acute lung injury (TRALI) is noted when used simultaneously along with the amphotericin B therapy

Q25. Which of the following is true regarding RING trial?
1. RING stands for Resolving Infection in Neutropenia with Granulocytes
2. The Trial assesses the individuals being treated for neutropenia, when administered granulocyte transfusions along with antimicrobial therapy, would have a higher likelihood of surviving to 42 days and attaining a microbial response, when compared to those receiving only antimicrobial therapy
3. The number of granulocytes in each granulocyte unit are evaluated with the goal of 4×10^{10} per collection (or correspondingly less for subjects under 30 kg)
4. All of the above

Q26. Which of the following is true regarding ProGrES (PROspective Granulocyte usage and outcomEs Survey)?
1. Granulocyte transfusions are considered for transfusion to patients with refractory infection who have quantitative or qualitative deficiencies of neutrophils
2. The study will focus on understanding how granulocytes are used in the UK
3. The study includes patient demographics, underlying conditions and treatment received, e.g. type of leukaemia, chemotherapy treatment, concomitant treatment for infection, indication for transfusion, dose and schedule, and outcomes
4. All of the above

Q27. A donor is undergoing granulocyte collection. Pre-apheresis granulocyte count (Pre-count): 30.0 × 10^9/L. Post-apheresis granulocyte count (post-count): 18.0 × 10^9 /L. The total blood volume processed is 3L excluding anticoagulant. The product has 154 × 10^9/L granulocytes with a bag volume of 250 ml. Calculate the collection efficiency:
1. 72%
2. 53%
3. 48%
4. 66%

ANSWERS

Q1. Ans(4)

Q2. Ans(4)

Granulocyte transfusion is not indicated for therapeutic use in:

1. Patients with bone marrow failure where neutrophil recovery is not anticipated to recur spontaneously and no further active treatment is planned
2. Sepsis occurs without neutropenia or known neutrophil dysfunction
3. Pyrexia of unknown origin (PUO)
4. Viral infection in the absence of additional proven or highly probable fungal or bacterial infection unresponsive to appropriate antimicrobial therapy.

Q3. Ans(4)

Malcolm Moore and Karl Welte isolated G-CSF from human cells in 1984. The function of G-CSF includes the differentiation of myeloid cell series from progenitor cells to mature neutrophil cells. The functions also include cell division, apoptosis, maturation, and phagocytosis of granulocytes.

Q4. Ans(4)

The CSF3 gene makes human G-CSF (hG-CSF), which is found on chromosome 17. There are 177 amino acids in G-CSF a and 174 amino acids in G-CSF b. G-CSF b have a glycosylation site on the oxygen called O-linked glycosylation., G-CSF b has nearly 20 times more biological activity compared to G-CSF a and hence it is preferred for commercial G-CSF preparations.

The granulocyte colony-stimulating factor receptor (homo dimeric G-CSFR) facilitates the function of G-CSF. GCSF-R found in all granulocytic cells, and in non-hematopoietic organs such as the, vascular endothelial cells, placenta, neural stem cells and cardiomyocytes.

Normal healthy individuals often have low levels of G-CSF which measures less than 100 pg/mL. When an individual is under stress or inflammation, the G-CSF levels elevate to 20 times the normal level. This in turn helps in rise of neutrophil count in blood.

Q5. Ans(4)

The differentiation of granulocytes is regulated by myeloid transcription factors such as PU.1, which belongs to the CCAT enhancer binding protein family, and GFI-1. Myeloperoxidase and serine proteases are present mainly in primary granules which are likely to emerge during the promyelocyte stage. The lactoferrin and collagenase are present in secondary granules, and gelatinase is found in tertiary granules; the secondary and tertiary granules are likely to develop during the myelocyte stage.

Q6. Ans(4)

The factors such as corticosteroids, physical activity, cytokines like G-CSF, chemokines, or substances from bacteria are known to trigger the possible quantity or amount of neutrophils produced and sent out from bone marrow to a great extent.

Q7. Ans(4)

Image: Fig-XIII-1: *In memoriam: Malcolm A.S. Moore (1944–2025)*. Leukemia. 2025 (Welte K)© The Author(s) This figure is reproduced from Welte K, Mertelsmann R. Licensed under Creative Commons Attribution 4.0 International (CC BY 4.0).

Dr. Moore was born in the United Kingdom in 1944 and obtained his doctorate from Oxford University in 1967. During his tenure, he was designated the youngest Prize Fellow of Magdalen College, Oxford.

His accomplishments involved purification and advancement of G-CSF, culminating in Filgrastim medication in the 1980s

The American Society of Clinical Oncology (ASCO) designated this discovery as a "Major Cancer Milestone." This medication elevates the production of white blood cells in individuals who have a low count due to chemotherapy and also strengthens the immune systems.

Q8. Ans(4)

Q9. Ans(4)

Q10. Ans(4)

Q11. Ans(4)

Q12. Ans(4)

Q13. Ans(4)

Q14. Ans(4)

Q15. Ans(4)

Q16. Ans(4)

Q17. Ans(4)

A study focussing on the removal of hydroxyethyl starch from donor blood indicated that it takes 72 weeks for serum levels to fall to baseline after multiple apheresis, while it takes 38 weeks after a single apheresis procedure. Given these challenges, the use of HES in healthy blood donors is ethically questioned and has prompted search for better and safer alternatives.

Q18. Ans(4)

The administration of HES is known to cause metabolic disturbances as hypernatremia, and can lead to neurological symptoms like confusion, seizures, or even coma. Hyperosmolar properties of few HES solutions are responsible for metabolic disturbances.

Q19. Ans(4)

A modified fluid gelatin (MFG) may be an alternative RBC sedimentation agent needed for granulocyte production. The biological half-life of MFG in the human body is 2.5 hours, shorter when compared to high-molecular-weight HES. The granulocyte yields are lower if MFG is used.

Q20. Ans(4)

Infusions should be given until one of the following events:

1. Clear evidence of endogenous recovery is observed, as indicated by the neutrophil count. The increase in

neutrophils resulting from granulocyte transfusions is unlikely to surpass 1.0×10^9/L. Consequently, it is prudent to proceed until the absolute neutrophil count exceeds 1.0×10^9/L on two consecutive days.

2. Resolution of infection occurs.

Q21. Ans(3)

Q22. Ans(4)

Volume: 200-400 ml, Concentration: 1×10^{10} granulocytes, Hematocrit: 50%±5%

Other granulocytes: 0.1-0.7 × 10^9

Platelets -2-10 × 10^{11}, Plasma- 100-300 ml

Q23. Ans(3)

Q24. Ans(4)

1. Transfusion-associated graft-versus-host disease (TA-GvHD). The granulocyte concentrate contains a significant amount of lymphocyte contamination, which inherently increases the risk of TA-GvHD. Consequently, granulocyte concentrates or pools must undergo irradiation before transfusion.
2. Transmission of infectious agents. The limited duration from collection to transfusion hinders the completion of standard laboratory testing for infectious diseases before the issuance and transfusion of the granulocyte concentrate. Additionally, leukoreduction is not recommended for granulocyte concentrates. Instances of granulocyte-related transmission of West Nile virus and cytomegalovirus (CMV) have been documented. To prevent CMV transmission, some suppliers or healthcare providers opt for CMV seronegative donors for recipients who are also CMV seronegative. Nevertheless, CMV seronegative products may not always be accessible.
3. Acute transfusion reactions. While most reactions are classified as mild, there have been serious complications that necessitated admission to an intensive care unit. In the RING trial, grade 1–2 reactions were observed in 41% of patients (including fever, chills, and/or slight changes in blood pressure). Grade 3–4 reactions (such as hypoxia, tachycardia, hypotension, and allergic symptoms) occurred after at least one transfusion in 20% of patients, although this represented less than 5% of all transfusions overall. No fatalities due to transfusion reactions were reported.
4. Acute pulmonary complications. In earlier decades, there were concerns regarding granulocyte transfusions in conjunction with the initiation of amphotericin B treatment, as a syndrome resembling transfusion-associated acute lung injury (TRALI) was noted in a report from the NIH. However, this association has not been confirmed in subsequent studies. Despite this, granulocyte transfusions are sometimes administered a few hours apart from amphotericin B treatment. It is not necessary to separate the administration of amphotericin B and granulocyte transfusion, and doing so should not delay the provision of either therapy.
5. HLA Alloimmunization. Granulocytes expose recipients to additional donor HLA antigens and may provoke HLA alloimmunization. Those receiving granulocyte transfusions have higher chances of developing alloimmune platelet refractoriness.

Q25. Ans(4)

The 2015 RING (Resolving Infection in Neutropenia with Granulocytes) study investigated the clinical effectiveness of granulocyte transfusion for established infections; it stands as the largest randomized controlled trial (RCT) of granulocyte transfusions to date, involving 14 participating centres, and was included in the Cochrane systematic review. The trial was halted prematurely due to insufficient enrolment, with only 114 patients recruited out of the targeted 236. The success rates (determined by the primary composite outcome of survival and infection resolution) for both granulocyte and control groups showed no significant differences across any infection type. A post-hoc analysis revealed better mortality outcomes in patients who received higher doses (>0.6 × 10^9 granulocytes/kg) compared to those who received lower doses. Nevertheless, since there was no significant difference between the high-dose treatment group and the control group, many consider this finding to be merely hypothesis-generating.

Q26. Ans(4)

This is a registry for the purpose of monitoring granulocyte transfusions, mainly concentrating on the usage, apart from focussing on treatment protocols, patient demographics and clinical outcomes and it is international. The study protocol sketches a prospective study which can assess the results following granulocyte transfusions in the UK. The study prefers to collect data on the indications, dosage, and results of granulocytes administered to both children and adults.

Q27. Ans(2)

%CE = Granulocyte count of bag × bag volume × 100/ (average of pre donation& post donation granulocyte count) × net volume processed

average of pre donation & post donation granulocyte count = 30.0×10^9 /L.+ 18.0×10^9 /L / 2 = 24.0×10^9 /L

Granulocyte count of bag × bag volume = $154 \times 10^9 \times 250$

$154 \times 10^9 \times 250 \times 100/24.0 \times 10^9$ /L × 3L = 53%

REFERENCES

1. S Morton & S Stanworth. INF276/5 Clinical Guidelines for the use of Granulocyte Transfusions. Blood and transplant NHS.2021
2. Link H. Current state and future opportunities in granulocyte colony-stimulating factor (G-CSF). Supportive Care in Cancer. 2022 Jun 24;30(9):7067–77.
3. Salazer E, Rice L. Neutrophil production and kinetics: neutropenia and neutrophilia: Simon TL, Gehrie EA, McCullough J, Roback JD, Snyder EL. Rossi's Principles of Transfusion Medicine.6th edition. Hoboken, NJ: John Wiley & Sons: 2022.
4. Khlusov I, Litvinova L, Efimenko A. Stem Cell Niche Concept: Search for Current Expert Consensus. International Journal of Molecular Sciences [Internet]. 2025 Aug 29 [cited 2025 Sep 18];26(17):8422. Available from: https://www.mdpi.com/1422-0067/26/17/8422
5. Petcova J, Goldberg C, McCullough J. Granulocyte collection and transfusion: Simon TL, Gehrie EA, McCullough J, Roback JD, Snyder EL. Rossi's Principles of Transfusion Medicine. 6th edition. Hoboken, NJ: John Wiley & Sons: 2022. p.194-99.
6. D.NO 1M11016/08/2025-NBTC/BTS DATED 10.12.2025 Government of India, Ministry of Health & family welfare, DGHS. (National Guidelines for Granulocyte Donations, Processing and Transfusion.)
7. Nanya, M., Yurugi, K., Kato, I. *et al.* Successful granulocyte apheresis using medium molecular weight hydroxyethyl starch. *Int J Hematol* 2019;110, 729–735.
8. Knapp S, Brosig A, Troeger A, Kleinschmidt K, Offner R, Selim Corbacioglu, et al. Granulocyte transfusions made with modified fluid gelatin in pediatric and adolescent patients with prolonged neutropenia. Transfusion. 2021 Dec 15;62(2):306–15.
9. https://profedu.blood.ca/en/transfusion/clinical-guide/granulocyte-transfusion-therapyChapter Granulocyte transfusion therapy Website: Canadian blood servicesAuthors: Erma Gardner MBChB, FCP(SA), Cert Clin Haem Phys (SA); Maria Fernandes, PhD; Catherine Latour MD, FRCPC; Matthew Seftel, MD, MPH, MRCP, FRCPC; Jason Acker, PhD, MBA; Gwen Clarke, MD, FRCPC
10. Price TH. The RING study: A Randomized Controlled Trial of GCSF-stimulated Granulocytes in Granulocytopenic Patients. Blood. 2014; 124(21):SCI-16-SCI-16
11. https://www.nhsbt.nhs.uk/clinical-trials-unit/trials-and-studies/blood-and-transfusion/progres/
12. Bryant BJ, Yau YY, Byrne PJ, Stroncek DF, Leitman SF. Gravity sedimentation ofgranulocytapheresis concentrates with hydroxyethyl starch efficiently removes red blood cellsand retains neutrophils. Transfusion. 2010 Jun;50(6):1203–9.
13. Welte K, Mertelsmann R. In memoriam: Malcolm A.S. Moore (1944–2025). Leukemia. 2025;39:3058. doi:10.1038/s41375-025-02806-0. Licensed under CC BY 4.0.
14. Pathak A, Panda D, Tejwani N, Mehta A. A study on beneficial impact of the use of medium-molecular-weight hydroxyethyl starch in granulocyte apheresis using continuous-flow cell separator Spectra Optia: A retrospective single-center study at a tertiary care oncology center. Asian J Transfus Sci. 2024; 18(1):79-84.
15. Myburgh JA, Finfer S, Bellomo R, Billot L, Cass A, Gattas D, et al. Hydroxyethyl starch or saline for fluid resuscitation in intensive care. N Engl J Med. 2012;367:1901–11.

Chapter 16

PLATELETPHERESIS

Dr. Indira S Puthran

Q1. The minimum platelet content per apheresis (single donor platelet) unit is:
1. 1×10^{11} platelets
2. 2×10^{11} platelets
3. 3×10^{11} platelets
4. 5×10^{11} platelets

Q2. According to Guidelines for blood donor selection and blood donor deferral 2025, after plateletpheresis donation, a donor should not be accepted for whole blood donation for at least _____days provided reinfusion is complete:
1. 1 day
2. 7 days
3. 14 days
4. 28 days

Q3. The maximum frequency of plateletpheresis donations permitted per month is typically:
1. 4 times
2. 2 times
3. 1 time
4. Unlimited

Q4. What is the usual minimum interval between two plateletpheresis donations?
1. 24 hours
2. 48 hours
3. 1 week
4. 2 weeks

Q5. The primary advantage of single-donor platelets over pooled platelets is:
1. Lower platelet yield
2. Increased donor exposure
3. Reduced alloimmunization risk
4. Lower cost

Q6. Which of the following is NOT a contraindication for plateletpheresis?
1. Citrate allergy
2. Unstable angina
3. Recent aspirin intake
4. Hemoglobin of 12.5gm/dl

Q7. The anticoagulant conventionally used in plateletpheresis is:
1. EDTA
2. Heparin
3. ACD-A
4. Sodium fluoride

Q8. Apheresis platelets should be stored with continuous agitation at:
1. 1–6 °C
2. 10- 20 °C
3. 20–24 °C
4. 30- 37 °C

Q9. Pre-donation platelet count is required:
1. Always before donation
2. If donation within 4 weeks
3. Never before donation
4. Only first donation

Q10. Minimum acceptable platelet pH at end of storage is:
1. >5.5
2. >6.0
3. >6.5
4. >7.0

Q11. Maximum number of plateletpheresis donations per week is:
1. 1
2. 2
3. 3
4. 4

Q12. Minimum baseline platelet count for plateletpheresis:
1. $100 \times 10^3/\mu L$
2. $120 \times 10^3/\mu L$
3. $150 \times 10^3/\mu L$
4. $200 \times 10^3/\mu L$

Q13. Which medication intake disqualifies a plateletpheresis donor?
1. Recent aspirin intake
2. Analgesics
3. Vitamins
4. Oral contraceptives

Q14. Which among the following is false regarding platelet collection by apheresis?
1. Platelets by apheresis were available since 1970
2. The apheresis can cause side effects as anemia, thrombocytopenia and lymphopenia in the donor
3. In 1988, the FDA declared that a donor can undergo plateletpheresis up to 24 procedures a year
4. None of the above

Q15. Correct management of syncope during plateletpheresis is:
1. Continue procedure
2. Increase flow rate
3. Discontinue procedure
4. Monitor the donor

Q16. Minimum donor weight for plateletpheresis is:
1. 45 kg
2. 50 kg
3. 55 kg
4. 60 kg

Q17. Primary function of platelet additive solution is to:
1. Increase platelet count
2. Reduce plasma reactions
3. Extend shelf life
4. Decrease pH

Q18. Minimum permissible volume of plateletpheresis product is:
1. 100 mL
2. 150 mL
3. 200 mL
4. 250 mL

Q19. Shelf life of platelet concentrate after irradiation is:
1. 24 hrs
2. Same as original expiry date
3. 7 days
4. 48 hours

Q20. Which donor parameter most strongly correlates with platelet yield?
1. Donor age
2. Donor height
3. Platelet count
4. Hemoglobin

Q21. Which is NOT a bacterial risk-reduction strategy for platelets?
1. Pathogen reduction
2. Bacterial culture
3. Platelet irradiation
4. Storage containers

Q22. Which factor does NOT limit platelet yield?
1. Poor venous access
2. Low hematocrit
3. Very high platelet count
4. Short procedure time

Q23. Most common donor reaction during apheresis is:
1. Syncope
2. Hematoma
3. Hemolysis
4. Citrate toxicity

Q24. Which does NOT prevent citrate toxicity?
1. Oral calcium
2. Symptom monitoring
3. Magnesium supplementation
4. Slower ACD infusion

Q25. Swirling in platelet QC indicates:
1. Artifact
2. Discoid morphology
3. Bacterial contamination
4. Poor quality

Q26. Higher hematocrit affects plateletpheresis yield by:
1. Reducing yield
2. Increasing yield
3. No effect
4. Improving separation

Q27. Typical anticoagulant-to-blood ratio in plateletpheresis is:
1. 1:1
2. 1:2
3. 1:10
4. 1:20

Q28. What is the standard irradiation dose for platelet component to prevent graft versus host disease?:
1. 5 Gy
2. 10 Gy
3. 25 Gy
4. 50 Gy

Q29. Expected platelet increment after one adult dose of single donor platelet is:

1. 5–10 $\times 10^3/\mu L$
2. 10–20 $\times 10^3/\mu L$
3. 20–40 $\times 10^3/\mu L$
4. 50–70 $\times 10^3/\mu L$

Q30. If products are leucocyte reduced, 95% of the units sampled must have residual leucocyte count below:

1. 3×10^6
2. 5×10^6
3. 10×10^6
4. 15×10^6

Q31. Interval between a whole blood donation and subsequent cytapheresis procedure shall be at least:

1. 2 weeks
2. 4 weeks
3. 6 weeks
4. 8 weeks

Q32. Which parameter is NOT routinely monitored during plateletpheresis?

1. Blood pressure
2. Heart rate
3. Oxygen saturation
4. Hypocalcemia symptoms

Q33. Maximum permissible time without agitation for platelets is:

1. 12 hrs
2. 24 hrs
3. 30 hrs
4. 48 hrs

Q34. Which factor is NOT routinely considered in donor selection?

1. HLA matching
2. Venous access
3. Hematology parameters
4. Drug history

Q35. In our plateletpheresis, we collected a product with a platelet concentration of 350×10^9 cells/unit. The donors' pre-count was 260,000/µL (260×10^9/L), and the post-count was 200×10^9/L. We processed a blood volume of 2000 mL without AC. What is the collection efficiency?

1. CE of a Platelet Collection is 76%; $350,000/((260,000 + 200,000)/2) \times 2)) \times 100 = 76.0\%$
2. CE of a Platelet Collection is 76.9%; $200,000/((260,000 /2) \times 2))) \times 100 = 76.9\%$
3. CE of a Platelet Collection is 74.2%; $260,000/(350,000/2) \times 2)) \times 100=74.2\%$
4. CE of a Platelet Collection is 57.14%; $200,000/((350,000 /2) \times 2))) \times 100 = 57.14\%$

ANSWERS

Q1. Ans(3)	Q2. Ans(2)	Q3. Ans(1)	Q4. Ans(2)	Q5. Ans(3)	Q6. Ans(4)
Q7. Ans(3)	Q8. Ans(3)	Q9. Ans(1)	Q10. Ans(2)	Q11. Ans(2)	Q12. Ans(3)
Q13. Ans(1)	Q14. Ans(4)	Q15. Ans(3)	Q16. Ans(2)	Q17. Ans(2)	Q18. Ans(3)
Q19. Ans(2)	Q20. Ans(3)	Q21. Ans(3)	Q22. Ans(3)	Q23. Ans(2)	Q24. Ans(3)
Q25. Ans(2)	Q26. Ans(1)	Q27. Ans(3)	Q28. Ans(3)	Q29. Ans(3)	Q30. Ans(2)
Q31. Ans(4)	Q32. Ans(3)	Q33. Ans(3)	Q34. Ans(1)	Q35. Ans(1)	

REFERENCES

1. National Blood Transfusion Council(NBTC) and Blood Transfusion Services Division. Transfusion Medicine Technical Manual. 3rd ed. New Delhi: Directorate General of Health Services, Ministry of Health and Family Welfare, Government of India; 2023.
2. Simon TL, Gehrie EA, McCullough J, Roback JD, Snyder EL, editors. Rossi's Principles of Transfusion Medicine. 6th ed: Wiley-Blackwell; 2022.
3. Vassallo RR, Winters JL. Apheresis : Principles and Practice. Vol. 2. Bethesda (MD; Bethesda, Maryland: AABB Press; 2021.
4. Kozanoglu I., *Problem Solving in Apheresis Medicine*, Switzerland:Springer Nature; 2024.
5. Andreu G, Vasse J, Sandid I, Tardivel R, Semana G. Use of random versus apheresis platelet concentrates. Transfusion Clin Biol. 2007;14(6):514–12.
6. Das SS, Chaudhary R, Verma SK, Ojha S, Khetan D. Pre- and post- donation haematological values in healthy donors undergoing plateletpheresis with five different systems. Blood Transfus. 2009;7(3):188–92.
7. Richa E, Krueger P, Burgstaler EA, Bryant SC, Winters JL. The effect of double- and triple-apheresis platelet product donation on apheresis donor platelet and white blood cell counts. Transfusion. 2008;48:1325–32.
8. American Association of Blood Banks. Standards for Blood Banks and Transfusion Services. 32nd ed. Bethesda (MD): AABB; 2020
9. Guidelines for Blood Donor Selection and Blood Donor Deferral issued by National Blood Transfusion Council, Director General of Health Services, Ministry of Health and Family Welfare, Government of India, New Delhi 2025

INDEX

A

B

C

D

E

F

G

U

V

W

Z

Disclaimer: The views and opinions expressed in the book are those of the authors and editors in their personal and professional capacity as medical educators. They do not reflect the official policy or position of any institute (Private/Government).

Medical Notice: Medicine is an everchanging science. Neither the Editors/ Authors nor the Publisher assumes any liability for any injury or damage resulting from the use of the material contained in this book. It is advised to follow the standard guidelines.

www.ingramcontent.com/pod-product-compliance
Lightning Source LLC
LaVergne TN
LVHW070953210926
848482LV00002B/204
* 9 7 9 8 9 0 3 6 2 3 3 9 6 *